rest.

T G Hancock

PAPERBACK

Cardiac Arrest.

© Copyright 2017

Thelma Hancock

The right of Thelma Hancock to be identified as author of this work has been asserted by her in accordance with the Copyright, Designs and Patents Act 1988.

All Rights Reserved.

No reproduction, copy or transmission of this publication may be made without written permission.

No paragraph of this publication may be reproduced, copied or transmitted save with the written permission of the publisher, or in accordance with the provisions of the Copyright Act 1956 (as amended).

Any person who commits any unauthorised act in relation to this publication may be liable to criminal prosecution and civil claims for damages.

While the story is set in Carlisle and its hospital, it is not, nor does it represent, any of the nursing and medical staff, who are figments of my imagination, as is the storyline. The wards are maintained excellently. Outbreaks of Norovirus happen in many hospitals and are dealt with expediently.

A CIP catalogue record for this title is available from the British Library.

ISBN 978-1-912462-09-4

eBook ISBN 978-1-912462-08-7

Printed and Bound in Great Britain

Chapter 1.

As Alexis gowned up she wondered where the man had gone; probably some father desperate to see his new born. She gave another small sigh. She was a cardiac nurse, but they were so short handed that the agency had sent her over to the Mother and Baby Unit anyway. She pulled on gloves as the wailing escalated, then was abruptly cut off.

Pushing open the door with a shoulder she came to an abrupt halt, standing glaring at the blue-eyed man who was rocking the child. At least he had an apron and mask now.

'What are you doing? Put that child down and get out of here. Norovirus is highly infectious. Can't you read?' She advanced into the room, her five foot three figure and thirty-six inch bust bristling and ready to defend her charges from ignorant fathers and would be paedophiles alike.

'Be quiet, woman. I've got her asleep. Your screeching is likely to wake the dead.' He gently laid the small bundle back into the cot, where a large burp signified the reason for the wailing in the first place.

'Screeching.' Alexis all but hissed the word. She scowled over her mask. 'I don't know who you are but you can't just wander about the ward dressed like that.' She pointed a gloved hand at the door. 'Out.' She glanced at the sleeping child and pointedly waited for him to leave the room.

Closing the door behind him she stripped off her gown and, tugging down the mask to loop under her chin, looked him over. 'What the hell do you think you're doing up here? She took a breath, 'And I don't screech.'

He undid his mask, dropping it into the bin next to the door. 'Well, no, perhaps not, you crooned quite beautifully to baby Jones when I saw you a few minutes ago. But this one had just dropped off and I had to stop you somehow.'

Alexis was opening her mouth for another withering retort as he finished disrobing. 'Must go. *Wela di.*' He leant over and dropped a feather light kiss on her lips effectively shutting her mouth.

He was half way down the corridor before she thought of a suitable answer, and dignity, as well as another piercing wail, prevented her from following up on the thought with a slap to the handsome cheek.

'Well really!' Which she felt was inadequate in the circumstances. She pushed the thought of the kiss away. She had work to do.

Her recent encounter was almost forgotten until the end of the shift when handover was in full swing. 'Did Josh find you, Alexis?'

'Who?'

The Staff Nurse shrugged, 'Doesn't matter, Mr Blevins, Cardiac consultant. He was up here earlier, wanted to know if we had enough staff. He's caring for Mrs Cresswell. I told him we'd got a couple of agency nurses filling the gap for a few days.' She offered a tired smile, 'When do we ever have enough staff?'

'Now, back to business. I'm of the opinion that we should move the Cresswell baby to the side ward. I'm not sure he will do.' The voice was impassive but the Staff's grey eyes reflected her sorrow. Baby Cresswell would be lucky to see the night out. She got a nod from the nurse in charge of him. 'I'll see to it now, if you've finished with me?'

'Off you go, Frieda.'

Alexis handed over her own workload with a sigh of relief and gathered her bag and denim jacket. She didn't want to be around when the Cresswell parents were informed. This was why she was a cardiac nurse. The patients tended to have had a life, at least, before they died.

ALEXIS WOULD HAVE BEEN surprised to know how well her thoughts matched those of Josh Blevins. He was sitting watching, through the top of the incubator, the incredibly tiny chest of baby Cresswell, as he struggled with each shallow breath. Dehydration on top of barely developed lungs was taking the life away from this baby minute by minute.

The mother was hardly fit to leave her bed but he'd gently suggested that she might be brought in to nurse her son for his final few hours. The doctors had done all they could. He would see if overwhelming love would make a difference.

He stroked the tiny hand with a glove encased forefinger and felt the tiniest of grips. His black brows twitched and the blue eyes developed a gleam. The eyes of the newborn remained tightly closed but there was a will to live in there, he was sure of it. 'OK, *Cariad*, if you do your bit we'll keep trying.' He whispered the words and then, without loosing the finger, sat back his infection control suiting rustling, and watched, waiting for the mother to be wheeled in.

He was thinking about that small grip as he walked off the ward, a few minutes later, it was such a small sign. Sometimes that was all he had to work with. Paediatric patients couldn't speak and tell him what was wrong. He had to trust his instincts and hope that he was reading them right. He walked outside the hospital and into the grounds, heading towards his four-wheel-drive. The Cherokee Jeep was silver and stood out among the MG's and BMW's like a cart horse among thoroughbreds, but he preferred its solid power to the more sporting models.

He swung aboard and started up, heading home for some tea and maybe a chance to take the weight off his feet. He was absorbed in thought about the last operation he'd performed that day but his lips moved into a fleeting smile, as a new thought presented itself. He hoped he wasn't about to be charged with sexual harassment, but instinct had dictated that kiss earlier in the day. His tongue poked out and gently ran over his lips. A very pleasant episode in a rather stressful day. He wondered what the young nurse was called. She seemed to have a way with the babies.

Alexis was walking home. She'd turned off the roadway and taken a short cut through and round the Carlisle castle. Its sandstone and mica reflected the spring sunshine after the rain had made the ground muddy underfoot. There was a green haze over the trees as buds burst into life and the smell of bluebells was wafting to her on a zephyr. She moved at a steady pace, keeping her eyes fixed on the ground in front of her, avoiding the potholes and doggy deposits, unaware of the admiring glances of males jogging past. She too was deep in thought.

'I shouldn't have allowed that kiss, but I didn't know he was going to do it did I?' She shook her head at a mallard rooting about, a stone's throw from the river Eden. 'I wonder what he said. It sounded foreign. I bet he was that Doctor.' She scowled at the next duck she passed. 'He should have told me who he was, but if he was, why didn't he gown up properly? Oh bother the man; I've got better things to do than worry about him.'

She was so deep in thought that she stepped out of Bitts Park, and off the pavement, and nearly under the four-by-four of the man she'd been thinking about. Josh had seen her in the distance, done a double take at the slim fitting jeans and the dark blue jacket, and noted the strawberry blonde hair loosened from its all enveloping cap then recaptured in a braid, but hadn't expected such a close-up of her face as it flashed in front of his windscreen.

He trod on the brake pedal and then forced himself to release his white knuckle grip of the steering wheel. He scrambled out of the driver's side, narrowly avoiding a car that had swerved behind and around him heading towards the roundabout ahead. 'Bloody hell!'

Alexis was stretched out in front of his radiator, her braid of hair flopped over her shoulder and both hands fisted into the ground. She turned her head as she heard a muttered litany of swear words and a stranger's hands running over her body with an expert touch.

'Don't you dare die on me, you hear, don't you bloody dare.'

'I'm not going to die. I'm sorry, I wasn't paying attention.'

'That much I got.'

Josh lifted her up and carried her to the passenger side door. 'Hospital. Let's have you checked out.'

The, up to present, quiescent bundle in his arms, began to struggle. 'No way, I'm a box of fluffies, honest, just a bit shook up.'

Josh shook his head. Even while he raised an eyebrow. 'Get in the car.'

'No.' She shook an emphatic head the plait swinging back and forward, 'I'm going home, no harm, no foul.' She took advantage of the slackening of his arms to slide down and stand on her own two feet. He stepped back as she brushed ineffectually at the mud on her clothes and then looked at him. 'I am sorry, and it was my fault.'

Josh looked her over. 'At least let me take you home, or failing that for a drink, I for one could do with something and you certainly look as though you need one too.'

Alexis shook her head. 'I'll be fine.' She stepped back and away from him. 'You mustn't drink and drive you know. They take that very seriously here.'

He began to say he hadn't meant alcohol, but she was walking away. 'Hey, are you going to sue me?'

Alexis swung around and looked at him. 'I said it was my fault.'

'I meant for the kiss.' He swung around the vehicle and climbed in before she could answer. The engine fired but he didn't pull away. Now why he thought, watching her retreating figure rounding the corner and heading across the Eden Bridge, had he reminded her of that kiss?

'Well really.' She muttered to herself as she heard the engine approach and then recede as Josh swung around the roundabout. She looked at the blue haze hanging over the road in the backwash of his dispersing exhaust. She realised that that was the second time she'd uttered the same meaningless phrase, in the wake of the same man's passing. 'Botheration. Thank God, I'm agency; I'll tell them I don't want to go there again.'

She walked towards the Stanwix area of the

Border town with more attention than usual and a slight limp. But the fates were conspiring against her. The agency rang that evening. 'Yes, they agreed, she had done four shifts but they'd like her to do another couple.' Alexis frowned down the phone line. 'I know two nurses are due back tomorrow. Why do you need me? I'm not really a paediatric nurse.'

The voice at the other end of the line sighed quietly, 'I know that very well, Staff Nurse Bowen, but you do have paediatric experience, and not many do. It's a specialised area. The drug dosages alone are a nightmare for some of the younger graduates.'

Alexis pulled a face. 'Very well, but I want my own discipline as soon as possible.' This time she heard the sigh of relief down the line.

'If you could perhaps do the late shift for the next two days...' the voice offered tentatively, 'I'll see what I can do.'

'Thank you.' She replaced the receiver and allowed herself a groan. She could see her reflection in the windowpane. The face that looked back at her was pale in comparison to her normal healthy glow. She had washed her face and changed her jeans for a pair of soft jog bottoms and some thick socks, but there wasn't much she could do about the grazing on her hands, one of which had a large scar across the palm. She examined them again in the light from the sinking sun.

Just why she didn't want to go back on that particular ward she wasn't going to admit to herself or anyone else. But, it wasn't altogether to do with working a discipline she hadn't trained for, and did involve the blue eyed man and his kiss.

'I'M SORRY, MR BLEVINS, but it wasn't unexpected.' Josh looked at the small corpse neatly shrouded and laid in the cot. 'I've got the mother in a side room, she's aware, but I thought you would want a word with her.' The staff nurse looked up at the dark suited man in front of her. She noted the frown as dark as the suit but also the sorrow in the blue eyes that had lost all their sparkle.

He gave a nod. 'Yes, I'll come and speak with her in a minute or two. The houseman pronounced?'

'Yes, sir.' The Staff Nurse backed away and left him with the small body.

Josh unwrapped and looked at the tiny face. Feeling the already cooling skin. He removed the shroud and placed his stethoscope on the chest, listening. He didn't doubt the houseman had called it right. But he'd been so sure this one would last until morning at least. He palpated the tiny stomach and ran a gentle hand settling the limbs straight again and covering up the face. He shook his head. 'Bugger,' it was said quietly. He straightened up and set his shoulders back, preparing to speak to the parents of baby Cresswell, aged five days, victim of a bug that shouldn't be anywhere near a hospital ward.

After the weeping mother had been settled back on a side ward he returned to the nursing station and prepared to write up notes. He sat staring into space; pen poised even when a mug of coffee was pushed near his elbow. He turned his head after a minute or two, 'I wish we could find the source. One of your nurses, she reminded me to wash my hands. We all need that reminder, Staff. This damn bug must be lurking somewhere. This is the third outbreak in a year, I'm told.'

The Staff Nurse nodded. What could she say? They had fumigated, changed curtains, sterilised bedding, everyone was more than conscious of the need for hand washing.

'I want the usual, the parents have agreed to a PM. I hate asking but we need to make sure of the strain of norovirus and the actual cause of death.'

'COD was dehydration wasn't it, sir?'

Josh shook his head, not in denial but with puzzlement, 'He was dehydrated despite all your best efforts, but I think the underdeveloped lungs administered the coup-de-grâce. We need confirmation for the coroner.' He checked his watch, 'Midnight, I need to get home, I'm operating tomorrow.'

Staff nodded again, watching as he wrote up his findings and orders for the mother. They didn't know much about this man. He didn't normally appear on the paediatric ward. What was known was that he loved the young patients and hated loosing them when he did have occasion to visit.

Rumour said he was married. But whether he had children himself was, apparently, a closely guarded secret. When he'd appeared on the ward six months ago the nursing fraternity had preened and applied lipstick, but he didn't appear to notice. This, she supposed, explained the rumour of marriage that had run riot around the ward for the first few weeks.

Her thoughts were interrupted by him putting the mug down and pushing back his chair. 'Thank you, good night, Staff; call me if you have any concerns with Mrs Cresswell.'

She watched him heading out the doors, tall, dark haired, and moving like an athlete. Well, she couldn't blame the nurses under her care, but she'd glimpsed the banked down anger when he looked at the corpse of baby Cresswell. She wouldn't like to get the wrong side of him.

ALEXIS WAS AWAKE AS well but it wasn't concern for the source of the outbreak. She was using Skype to speak to a small child who was bouncing about on her foster mother's knee, touching the screen and leaning forward every so often to kiss it leaving slightly sticky marks which neither woman remarked.

'uv oo, 'exy.'

'I love you too, darling. He's been good?'

'He's always good, Alexis.' Her foster mother smiled. 'Not long now before you come home. It's done you good. I can tell from here.'

'I miss you both.'

'Well, we miss you, don't we, pet?'

The child, his small face alight with a beaming smile was understood to say that he missed Alexis too.

'You needed this time away. We can cope fine

here, just don't forget us.'

'As if I could. I owe you so much, Mother Mary.'

Her adopted mother grinned at her.

'It's time Peter was in bed and you got some rest.'

'Yes, I know, but he's restless tonight. I think it might be a tooth. I'll catch a bit of sleep tomorrow when he's at playgroup.'

'Huh! That'll be the day.' Alexis shook her head; 'You're as bad as he is.'

Mary Down shook her greying curls and shrugged shoulders clad in a thick fleece dressing gown, 'I love my charges. What's a bit of lost sleep if they can find happiness?'

Alexis, who had personal knowledge of how much sleep Mary had lost over the years, offered a lop-sided smile. 'Yeah, alright, I hear you.' She touched her lips to her fingers and then to the screen, 'Love you both. Goodnight.'

'Goodnight, love.'

Alexis switched off the small laptop and shut the lid slowly. She had just intended to leave a message on Facebook, but Mary was updating her status so had swapped to Skype when she'd seen the connection. It was good to catch up; Mary Down had been her mother in everything but birth since Alexis had been a terrified and miserable ten-year-old.

JOSH BLEVINS WAS LEANING over the bed of his five-year-old daughter. She was sound asleep, her pudgy hands clutching an old t-shirt of his, of grey and tattered aspect, it smelt of his aftershave. He smiled and moved closer, dropping a kiss on the thin cheek. Then sighed; he needed to get to bed, he was tired and he had an early surgery, but that wasn't the reason for the sigh.

He thought of the grief-stricken woman he'd left behind at the hospital. Her baby had been longed for, wanted desperately, and it had died. She wouldn't get another chance; the pregnancy had put her at severe risk. Her heart was barely strong enough to begin another pregnancy and carry another child to term. He was so lucky to have his little Emma.

He crept out of the room and got ready for bed, settling into his own king size and trying to relax his limbs. He didn't like bringing his work home, but sometimes it followed him.

He turned over and put the light out. He would think of, he mentally paused, he would think of the young nurse singing to the baby, ignoring the sickly smells, and the wails, just nursing it regardless. She obviously loved her job. He smiled in the dark as the image of her indignant face appeared on his mental screen and his tongue came out and licked over his lips in an absent way. A pretty thing, and she tasted good too. He drifted off, to dream of pink clouds and teddy bears and woke to find his daughter sitting on his chest talking to her teddy as she rocked it.

'Hello, *Cariad*, how are you today?'

His daughter gave him a gap-toothed smile her tongue poking out a bit over the words. 'OK, daddy.' Her slanted brown eyes, so typical of Downs' children, sparkled with pleasure.

'Do you want a little *cwtch* or a big *cwtch*? Only dad has to go to work,' he looked at his watch, 'very, very soon.'

'Big.' The small body, in the all in one pink suit, wormed under the duvet and an arm half strangled him. Teddy gave him a passing thump on the nose as he was dragged under the covers too. He received half a dozen kisses, each punctuated by a number.

'You're getting so good at counting.' He hugged back then swung out of bed with her in his arms. 'Its bath-time for you, young lady. Maria.' The bellow stirred the dust motes in the sunshine, and a young woman appeared at the door.

'Sorry, Dottore, I was just...'

'That's OK; here take her away, I must get ready. Bye-bye, *Cariad,* I'll see you later.'

Emma was borne away in her nanny's arms for a bath and dressing, and Josh prepared to deal with his own toilet in the en-suite. He was drying his hair with a large and fluffy towel in the bathroom, when his housekeeper, Joan, knocked on the bedroom door and called out, 'Tea, Josh, see you drink it!'

He scowled at the misty mirror and continued to dry himself off. He had employed Joan when he first became a father, but the relationship went back a lot further. She and her husband had looked after his elderly parents until their deaths a few years ago. Now they cared for him and his home.

He ate his breakfast at the big deal table in the sunny kitchen while he looked over the post, sorting it into private and work related. Taking periodical sips of coffee, and munching toast in between times.

Walking through to his study he dropped the private mail on his desk in an untidy heap and stuffed the others into his briefcase, then prepared to go and do battle with another day. His daughter was waiting at the front door for her kiss. Maria, her nanny, was hovering in the background; he glanced at her, 'No problems?'

'Little short of breath, Dottore. Not serious, and she used spacer.'

'Good.' He bent down and kissed the cheek offered. 'You be good for Maria and I might bring you a present.'

The chubby hands clapped and the bright brown eyes crinkled. 'Dolly?'

'Another one?' He scowled fiercely at her and she broke into giggles. He carried her happiness away with him as he got into the car and drove to work. His daughter would be very lucky if she made it to her next birthday. Her medical problems were legion. A dolly was little enough to give her.

ALEXIS ARRIVED ON THE ward at three o'clock, having enjoyed the luxury of a late breakfast and a trip to the shops before she reported for duty. The ward wasn't quite as frantic this afternoon.

'I'll give you the Jones' baby again, Staff, and if you could keep an eye on Samantha, and Kevin, but they seem to be almost out of the woods now. They've both kept their bottles down today. Fingers crossed.' The afternoon Staff Nurse, nodded at Alexis, 'Little Alun Jones is still very poorly. We've increased the fluids and he's been written up for some potassium. Get Frieda to check it out with you before she goes off, and she'll fill you in on anything else you need to know.'

The attention shifted to another nurse and her workload. Alexis listened carefully and took notes, nevertheless; she might have need to go to those children during the course of the shift.

They all stood up at the end of handover and she went off to look in on each of her charges, gowning and disrobing at each door afterwards. She wondered if she would see the Doctor again. She found she was thinking of him in inverted comma as 'the Doctor' and tried to remember what his first name had been. Had she heard it? She could remember his eyes, bright blue, and they'd crinkled at the corners. He'd had a nice tan too.

She shook her head, which was once again clothed in a paper cap with teddies running riot over it matching the gowns they all wore, but it didn't mask the serious nature of the job they were doing. Nothing could. What was she doing thinking of men? She had a good career; she wasn't going to be here much longer.

Six months she'd promised Mary, and then she would go home and help look after the other children. Mary had said it didn't matter, but it did, she owed her.

She was changing Samantha's nappy, and grateful for the mask she was still wearing, when she heard the smoke alarms. She flicked, snapped and wrapped in double quick time, tucking the small girl under her arm as going for the touch in a rugby game and going to the door. She opened it and sniffed. Sometimes the steriliser or the showers set the alarms off.

The Staff Nurse was standing in the corridor with the phone in her hands, talking rapidly. Alexis noted the other nurses standing either in doorways as she was, or at the desk all seemingly frozen in place. The Staff gave a final nod and then raised her voice, 'Hold your positions, there's a small fire in the A&E, someone set fire to a rubbish bin, probably a carelessly disposed cigarette. The Fire Brigade have been called. If we have to evacuate it will be to points A and D. Then, and only then, put the babies in hooded cots and wheel them down to the service elevators. Clear?'

Everyone murmured their agreement and understanding. Alexis stepped back and put Samantha down in her cot. She rapidly changed from one lot of protective gear to another and went over to Kevin's room. He had woken with the noise and was grizzling. She re-wrapped him and checked she had the hood handy before moving off to little Alun Jones.

Alun wasn't crying, and that was a worry. She

felt the tiny head, resting her fingers on the fontanel and marking the pulse. It was slower and more irregular than normal.

She leaned over pressing the button. 'OK, Munchkin, we're here now, don't you fret. She checked the fluid intake and nodded to herself as she slowed it down. Staff appeared at her elbow holding a mask to her mouth, wearing and apron but nevertheless leaning back so that she didn't contaminate the area. 'What's the problem?' She pitched her voice without shouting and distressing the baby.

'I suspect potassium or fluid overload; he's going into mild shock.'

'I'll page the houseman. 'She looked at the small silent boy in the cot. 'You've slowed it?'

'Yes. Right down.'

'Good.' She was already going out of the door, her words wafting back to Alexis as she disrobed, 'I'll reassign in case we have to evacuate.' She raised her voice yet more to reach above the noise of the alarm which was ringing in everyone's ears.

Alexis kept one eye on the slowly dripping IV line and the other on the child, while her fingers rested gently on the head, monitoring the heart-rate.

Her concentration was such that she visibly jumped when the houseman, a cheerful man by the name of Ben, who looked as though he'd be more at home on the rugby field, poked his head around the door, holding his mask against his mouth and keeping the rest of his body shielded by the woodwork. 'Settled? Need me to check him over? Or do you just want the fluids rewriting?'

'I think you'd better have a look. He's not sweating as much but the pulse is still a bit erratic.'

He withdrew his head and she could hear him speaking to someone outside. The stranger of the night before then shouldered the door aside, fully gowned and masked. 'I'll check him over for you, nurse; Ben's got enough on his plate, with panicking mothers and wailing babies. Oh! Thank God for that.' He shook his own head as the alarm was abruptly silenced and people, who had been shouting at each other outside the room, suddenly found themselves with loud voices and no reason for them.

'Now, young man, what have you been up to? He flipped his stethoscope from his neck set it in his ears and moved the small vest aside to examine the chest. Not that he needed to listen; the heartbeat was visible through the milky-white skin. The tiny blue veins tracking over the upper chest. He held the stethoscope a second or two in his palm before placing it against the beat. And frowned down as he concentrated on the valves opening and shutting, the soft whoosh of blood filling and ejecting, and the lungs labouring slightly. 'Mmm.'

He re-wrapped and smoothed the clothing down over the frail body. 'I'll need to take an ECG. Just to check on the t and p waves, but I think you've got to him in time, nice catch.'

'I can do the ECG,' Alexis raised an eyebrow

when he continued to frown at her. She added 'sir,' in case he was one of those consultants who thought themselves little gods. She frowned herself, her nicely shaped eyebrows meeting over her hazel eyes.

'Children's ECG's are a bit tricky, nurse.'

'Yes, sir.' Alexis drew her brows together even more, suppressing her indignation.

'I want a twelve lead and he's not got much chest. Sure you know what you're doing?'

Yes, sir.' This time he picked up on the slightly indignant tone.

'Right, I'll be back in ten minutes.' He nodded and swept out.

Alexis looked at the swinging door and pressed the call button. The Staff Nurse appeared in the entrance almost immediately, pushing the ECG machine in front of her. 'Here you go. Josh said you needed this. How's he doing, poor little mite?' She stopped before she'd taken more than a step inside.

'Steadying.'

'Need help?' Since she was already turning away as she said it Alexis shook her head,

'I'll be fine.' She switched on the machine and started to unravel leads. Muttering to herself and the baby in the cot. 'What did he expect, Alun. That you'd be a size forty-four chest with a six pack to match? You're only seven days old in heaven's name.'

She pulled out and began to position the paediatric pads around the small chest area, arms and legs, and was just checking everything over when Josh walked back in. 'OK.'

Alexis repressed the 'tut' of annoyance hovering on her tongue and nodded at him. She flicked the switch and watched the machine clicking its way through the analysis. Checking the printout, she nodded to herself, and began to take off the stickers, careful to ease them off the delicate skin. Josh, who stood next to the bed, silently watching her, waited patiently for her to finish making the child comfortable. He too had looked at the printout and smiled to himself under his mask.

'Tell me what the results are?'

Alexis glanced at him, still busy with the child. 'The print-out is there, sir.'

'I'm well aware of that, nurse. I want you to tell me what you saw.'

Alexis looked at him and then took the sheet of paper. "'T' wave is slightly peaked, spacing is only marginally extended, and the sheet shows typical mild overload of 'K', sir. He doesn't show any sign of depression of the pacemaker, the SA and AV nodes are normal. No widening or flattening. He's in sinus rhythm again. She added another, 'Sir.' with a slight snap.

He gave a nod. 'And you would recommend?'

'British nurses are not allowed to diagnose or prescribe.' She nodded at him and then recited, 'Unless they are nurse practitioners in a specialist field, sir.'

'Nevertheless, nurse, and don't recite rules

and regulations to me, I want to know what you see and recommend.'

Alexis smoothed the small white face and smiled, as Alun nuzzled her hand, before she turned to face Josh. 'Very well, sir, he is holding his own now, he isn't in need of the 'K', or if he is, only a much reduced amount, his kidney function should be checked to verify, but I would say reduce IV input and increase bottle feeds.'

'So would I, nurse.' He nodded at her, 'And for Christ's sake stop calling me, 'sir'. I don't know where you trained, but you're wasted on this ward and I want you on my team over in cardiac.'

Alexis shook her head at him, but before she could say another word he'd left the room with a decided swish of robes pulling down the mask as he exited.

She swallowed the, 'Really,' she had hovering on her tongue; she hadn't known she used the phrase so much. The man might be a consultant but he would find he couldn't order her around. She shook her head at her thoughts. Who was she kidding? She wanted Cardiac and he was offering it. He'd get a shock when he found out she was only Agency and not available for his team.

She smiled grimly and went off to check on her other charges, satisfied that Alun was settling nicely and would be yelling for a bottle very shortly.

Chapter 2.

JOSH MIGHT HAVE DESIGNS on Alexis as a nurse for his team, but he had other concerns to deal with this afternoon. It had been pure chance that saw him on the mother and baby ward at the time the Jones baby needed him.

He had come up to look in on Mrs Cresswell. She had been his patient before pregnancy and, while he had concerns about her health during that pregnancy, his primary concern now was preventing her overwhelming grief from doing what the birth hadn't, killing her.

He wrote his findings in Alun Jones' notes, penned the new instructions, signed the book with his scrawl, stood up and went to find his patient.

'Mrs Cresswell, Jane,' he gave the gentle smile reserved for his patients, as he shut the door on the single room to which he'd had her allocated. 'How's the tummy?'

'Worthless, I went through all that and all I've got is this...' she began to cry, harsh, hard, wrenching, sobs which turned eyes already red into liquid pools. Her brown curls stuck to her cheeks as they tracked down and her husband sitting in the hard chair near the bed reached for her hand and took a firm grip, but said nothing.

Josh sat carefully on the side of the coverlet and offered a tissue from the box on the over-bed table. 'I can't offer you any consolation, my dear. I know how hard you fought to conceive and carry. Another pregnancy might kill you.' He spoke gently but bluntly. 'You must not get pregnant again, the mitral valve cannot be repaired again, 'Any more strain and your next option will be a transplant.'

'I don't care. I want my baby!' The words were sobbed out.

Josh nodded, 'Yes. I know. But nothing could save him, even if he hadn't contracted norovirus. He would have been a very poorly little chap for most of his life, you were only twenty-three weeks. His chances were slim. Even in intensive care.' He paused, he didn't believe in soft peddling. Most people wanted the truth, he'd found.

'Take your time, get well, allow yourself to grieve,' he looked at her silent husband, 'both of you. You have another three or four days in hospital to recover from the birth, would you like me to have you transferred to a general surgical ward away from the noise here.'

Everyone in the room knew he meant the sound of babies crying but no-one said so.

Jane Creswell shook her head. 'I don't care.' She shredded the tissue in her hands and looked at him from those reddened and tear-drenched eyes. Her face grey from illness and emotion.

'Jock?'

'No, the noise is a bit of comfort, I think. Can you understand?'

'Yes, but if it gets too much you have only to say.' He laid a gentle hand on her shoulder and gave a squeeze, then turned and shook hands with Jock Cresswell. He left them both, shutting the door after himself. He went off down the ward and stopped briefly at the desk to speak to Gill, the Staff Nurse. 'She'll stay, with the option of going down to medical if need be; they've got a couple of spare beds at the moment. If the distress becomes too much, sedate. I've written her up for something.'

He turned on his heel and strode out of the ward down to the day-care ward where he'd performed several stents that morning. He put the sad scene to the back of his mind as he prepared to deal with his other patients.

The room was wide, with occupied beds spaced around the edges. His consulting rooms were just to the side of it. He cast an all encompassing look around, noting the presence of his staff, busy with paperwork for the most part this afternoon. Some patients dozed; most looked at him expectantly with the hope of going home plain on their faces.

'Any problems?'

The senior nurse looked up from her computer, her blonde hair coming down from the grip at the back, and her make-up at this time of day almost none existent on her pretty face. 'No, Josh. Do you want to do a round?'

'Yes.' He walked over and washed his hands, before approaching the bed of an elderly and very obese gent. 'How do you feel now, Mr Walker?'

Mr Walker looked at the handsome man in front of him and smiled. His eyes, surrounded as they were in wrinkles of fat, and jowls wagging at each word, spoke up in the voice of a man used to forty a day. 'Sore, but actually quite well, not breathless at all really.'

'Let's have a look at the site.' He waited for the curtains to go around and then looked at the small puncture wound in the right femoral artery. The icepack and sandbags that had helped the blood to congeal over the site had been removed and the wound was clean and dry.

'Had your sandwiches?'

Mr Walker nodded happily.

'Good, get the paperwork done, Staff.' He looked back at the elderly man. 'You can go home, see me in six weeks. I expect you to keep to your diet now, and don't undo all my good work.'

'No fear, you've given me a new lease of life. I'm not going to wreck it.'

'Good, you've got all you need, and you understand that you shouldn't lift or pull for a couple of weeks. Showers not baths, and take care.'

'You're the boss.'

Mr Walker still needed to lose seven or eight stone; but his efforts to lose five had been rewarded by Josh agreeing to perform the operation.

Josh went from bed to bed, going through much the same spiel, checking the wounds and sending people home. The invention of the stent had saved more lives than he could count. A piece of metal that resembled nothing more than the bent spring from a ballpoint pen inserted into a clogged vein, opening it up and allowing the heart to have a proper supply of blood and oxygen, was to his mind, a brilliant invention on a par with dynamite.

He went into his office and started on the mountain of notes for that day's procedures. Arthur Hardy, another patient, had had a minor infarction while they had been busy. The insertion of the lines that would deliver the stent to veins at the bottom of the right atrium had irritated the heart. Josh had had to abort the procedure on him, but he'd had Hardy warded. He'd check the latest ECG and maybe reschedule for the following week if nothing else occurred.

Various other patients' notes appeared, even as he worked on the one's already on his desk. There was the susurration of men and women leaving the ward speaking quietly, or with excitement, to their relatives. The sound of footsteps, some tentative, others quite springy, as the men and women under his care realised that the procedure they had come in for that morning, really was going to be, not just a life saver, but a life changer.

As the hours slid by, and the notes moved from one side of the desk to the other, the ward fell quiet. Josh became aware of the ticking of the clock and the nurses talking to each other. Once a giggle that he knew belonged to his much respected and normally sober head staff nurse, April. A bit later there was an enormous clang as someone dropped a large metal object that rang like a bell and echoed around the sterilisation room where the autoclave was working overtime. Eventually even these noises faded away.

He re-capped the old-fashioned pen his parents had given him when he passed his finals with a faint smile for the memory that always evoked.

April came in as he tucked it away. 'All set, Josh. Do you want a drink of coffee before I go?

'No, I'm good for now.' He sat back, swinging from side to side in the work chair. 'What do you know about a young nurse working up on paeds just now? Her name is Alexis; I'd say she's about 23, blonde hair in a braid, hazel eyes, sharp mind, and an equally sharp tongue.'

April raised eyebrows almost plucked to extinction. 'Heavens, Josh, what on earth...?' She stopped, she wasn't that sure of their relationship; he'd never invited or asked a personal question in the six months they'd worked together. Was he eyeing up a member of staff? If so it was a first.

He offered a lop-sided smile and patted the air. 'No. Nothing like that, April. But she showed extraordinary promise. I could use another skilled pair of hands on cardiac, I'd like to poach her.'

'And does she want to be poached?'

Josh wrinkled a nice straight nose and then grinned properly. 'I have no idea.' He gave a cough of laughter and April smiled broadly.

'I don't actually know who this Alexis is, but I'll have a word with Gill for you. She could maybe put out a few feelers.'

She watched as he frowned. 'I may have already put my foot in it. I told her she was wasted there and I wanted her.'

'I don't know about poaching, you are so fried, you're not that...' she hesitated, tucking her tongue metaphorically in her cheek, 'emancipated.' She suggested as he looked at her.

'No, probably not. See what you can do for me will you, there's a darling.'

April raised an eyebrow, Josh seemed different today. More, she watched as he stood up swinging over his shoulders the jacket that matched his nice suit trousers, relaxed.

'Its getting warm and it's only May.' He spoke apparently irrelevantly.

'Nearly June, then all the staff will be demanding holiday leave, even the ones who haven't booked any. And looking to me to bribe the surgeon into giving them it.' April grinned.

They exchanged smiles and Josh held the door open for her as he prepared to leave the day-ward. 'Call me if there are problems.'

He set off briskly down the corridor, heading for the main cardiac ward. He would check on Arthur

Hardy before he left for the evening.

Arthur Hardy was half-sitting half-lying in bed, his O_2 mask hissing quietly on the coverlet. He smiled as he saw Josh approaching down the four bed ward. 'Doc. Come to send me 'ome?'

'Hello, Mr Hardy. How do you feel now?'

'M leg's a bit sore, 'n so is this arm but 'm OK otherwise.'

Josh looked at the cannula running a saline drip at 20 drops a minute. He'd inserted it himself and he could see the site wasn't inflamed, but there was a bit of bruising around the area. 'We'll just finish up that bag, and then see how you go. I want you on bed rest for a couple of days. That's going to be annoying for you.' He sat down by the side of the whip-thin man and took a wrist, checking the pulse.

'You'll feel alright and want to get up, but I don't want you to. Ring the bell; the nurses will bring you a bottle or commode. They understand that you aren't being idle. It's important that you rest. You are to have small meals, six of them, instead of three big ones each day.'

'Aw, Doc, I'm fine now, no pain, not giddy, don't feel faint.'

'Let's keep it that way.'

'But, Doc, what'll the wife say? 'N me lollygagging 'ere, while she has to run the shop.'

Josh shook his head. 'I have rung your wife and explained that we're keeping you in for a few days. Understand this; if you keep going the way you have been, she will have to run your shop as a widow. You are not a well man. You are not...' He paused, "lollygagging', and that's a hell of a word, Mr Hardy. You have clogged arteries and an enlarged heart, your blood pressure is far too high, I want you both to celebrate your golden wedding next year, and if you don't rest you won't.'

'Well that's blunt enough. What did my Eddie say to you?' Arthur Hardy resettled himself against the bank of pillows. 'She thinks only fat blokes can have high blood pressure.'

'She took a little persuading, but I think we have come to an understanding now. High blood pressure is prevalent among the obese, but it's more a case of clogged arteries and fat around the main organs, and yours are loaded. You need to change your whole lifestyle. Both of you. And so I told her.' He smiled at Mr Hardy. 'She needs to lose a few pounds too; if you do it together it will be much easier.'

'My Gawd, Doc! I wish I could've listened in to that.'

'It's probably just as well you didn't; I want your blood pressure down.' He grinned at the grinning man next to him. 'OK, do we understand each other?'

'Yes, Doc, and thanks.'

'Right, I'll see you in a couple of days and reschedule your stent for next week.' Josh stood up, shook hands and headed off the ward, the smile still lingering on his face. It lightened the load to have had even partial success with a patient and he needed that load lightening today for some reason.

ALEXIS, MEANWHILE, WAS FEEDING a hungry baby two ml of milky water. Alun Jones had definitely turned the corner. He hadn't, it was true, taken kindly to having his blood taken, but once that ordeal was over he had snuggled down in her arms and was sucking slowly at the teat. 'You'll be able to have some of mum's milk soon, young man, and won't she be relieved. Her milk is in and she wants to give it to you. She's coming to give you a cuddle in a bit.' Alexis gave an expert twirl on the teat in his mouth, encouraging him to take the final drops. 'What a good boy.' Alun's eyes were already drooping. She carefully wrapped him and settled him in the cot, easing a light blanket over his body.

Having checked on her other charges she went over to a desk standing like the prow of a ship in the middle of the ward. She walked around and sat on one of the office chairs to write up fluid balances and, while she was there, eased off her grey clogs, resting her feet on the cool ground for a minute or two.

She was just signing her name when Gill, the Staff Nurse, came and sat next to her. 'I thought we'd seen the last of you.' She smiled, 'Not that you haven't been a Godsend, Alexis.'

'Tonight and tomorrow, and then its where the agency sends me next.' Alexis leaned back in the chair and pushed her hair over her shoulder. 'I think I'm going to take a couple of days off. It's the weekend coming up and the weather man promised two sunny days. You can't afford to ignore them.'

'Too right.'

Alexis gave her an odd look. 'Sometimes you sound more Aussie than English.'

'I've just been insulted. I'll have you know I'm a true blue Kiwi I am. Trained at Christchurch.'

Alexis beamed; there was no other word for it. 'My dad was a Kiwi; I lived in Christchurch for nearly eight years.'

'And you came over here! Are you mad?'

'Makes two of us; horrid weather, and so many people. Have you noticed how if you say you're a Kiwi they think you should know their relatives over there?'

'Weird isn't it?' They were laughing together when April came through the swing doors and leaned on the desk.

'Hi, Gill, heard you're starting to get topsides of the bug.'

'Yes,' Gill sighed deeply; 'it's been a bugger, April. I wish we knew the source. I don't know what else to do. I worry about the new babies on the ward every day.'

'Yeah, that I can understand.' She smiled in sympathy. 'Any chance of coming for a cuppa?'

'Nah! Can't leave at the moment, just taking five.'

April shrugged. 'Never mind.'

Alexis looked at the two women and got to her feet, shuffling them back into the clogs. 'I'd better get back to work.'

Both of them gave her a friendly smile as she rounded the desk and walked off. 'New member of the team?'

'Agency. Half the staff have had the norovirus; they're trickling back now, thank heavens. I've got notices up everywhere telling them to wash their hands. As if having the bug hasn't been warning enough.

April gave a half cough of laughter at the wry words, then came and sat down next to her friend in Alexis' previous seat. 'My boss wants to poach one of your team.'

'Oh yeah, which one.'

'Someone called Alexis.'

'He'll be lucky. She's just walked away from us, and she's agency.' Gill grinned. 'She is good, mind, fast worker, spots things before they've hardly started, great with the babies, like she's handled more than her fair share.'

'Is she paediatric trained then?'

'Suppose so, otherwise why send her to us.'

April shrugged. 'Well Josh said she; now let me get it right, she showed 'extraordinary promise.'' She bracketed the words in the air above her head.

'Oh, she's a bright cookie alright. I don't like agency normally; they can be more trouble than they are worth. By the time you've shown them where everything is, and maybe assigned one of the others to help them; you might as well not have the extra pair of hands. But she came on ward, spent ten minutes looking around and then just got on with it. And her notes are exemplary.'

April's mouth dropped open. She knew her friend's views about agency nurses and this was praise of no common order. 'Are you going soft in your old age?'

'Bloody cheek.' Gill gave her friend a pretend thump. 'So what do you want me to do?'

'Can't do much, he can't poach her off you anyway. Give me the name of the agency and I'll pass it on.'

Gill scrawled the name on her notepad and tore out the page. 'I must get on; the rest of them will call me a slacker.' She smiled at her friend. 'I've got Saturday evening; how do you fancy going to the cinema?'

'Yeah, alright, I shall deny all my boyfriends in favour of you.'

'Aw, sweet.' Gill grinned and stood up. 'Do you want me to say anything to Alexis?'

'Better not. Josh likes to keep things close to his chest.'

'I wonder if he does.'

'Eh!' April frowned at her friend as she started to walk away,

'Keep things close to his chest, like women?'

'That would be telling, and I don't tell, 'cos, a. I want to keep my job, and b.' she offered another grin as she walked away, 'I don't know.'

ALEXIS HEARD THE TWO women laughing as April walked away, and wondered what they'd been talking about. Then dismissed them as she concentrated on adjusting the naso-gastric tube of one of a pair of twins; he had a cleft palate and was struggling to suck. The consultant paediatrician had scheduled the operation for the next day. The twins lay in a double cot and she had been first astonished, and then charmed, to find them apparently holding hands.

She began to attend to their small wants; changing nappies and wiping small bottoms. Their mother would be in very shortly; she had another pair of twins at home and was dividing her time between the lot of them.

Alexis allowed her mind to wander slightly while she dealt with mundane tasks. It would be nice to go to the seaside. She missed the sea. Mother Mary's home was in Whitehaven, too far to commute, but not too far for a weekend visit. She needed to see a familiar face as much as the twins she'd just been dealing with.

When Alexis's father died her own mother had returned to her roots in England. Alexis had only just begun to find her feet in the small Yorkshire town where her kiwi accent caused comment. Then everything had changed; her mother had died in her sleep. A ten-year-old Alexis had discovered the body. Her mother had only been thirty-three. She'd died of Sudden Cardiac Death according to her death certificate; Alexis thought she'd died of a broken heart.

Alexis had waited for her mother to wake up for several hours that weekend, before she'd gone into her mother's bedroom and found her body. She'd had the sense to ring for an ambulance, but then life had gone downhill. Foster home had followed foster home. It seemed as if no-one wanted to adopt a ten-year-old with some serious hang-ups; until Mother Mary.

Alexis smiled as she crooned to the babies and tucked them securely into the cot. She set the pink and blue teddy bears straight at the end of the mattress and then turned to go out of the room with a quick glance at her fob watch.

Nodding at Gill, seated at the central console that she was taking her assigned break, she gathered up a cardigan and pulled it over her green scrubs. 'Back in a bit.'

Gill gave a nod in return as she signed yet another piece of paper.

Alexis made her way along the corridor and waited next to a pair of lifts, heading down to the staff canteen. The lift, when it arrived was large, big enough to accommodate a single bed with patient, a pair of porters; not to mention a midwife and a drip stand, and this was, in fact, was what met her eye when the doors wheezed their way open. The overwhelming smell of birth fluids blotted out, momentarily, the smell of disinfectant. Alexis smiled at the midwife and shook her head. 'I'll take the stairs.'

She watched in sympathy as the doors shut again; the mother-to-be was heading down for surgery; a difficult labour evidently; a deep groan could be heard just before the doors finally shut them back in on their downward journey. She stepped back smartly and was about to turn and head for the stairwell when the second lift shuddered to a stop and, with a ping, opened its doors. This time the smell that teased at her nostrils was aftershave. Very clean and faintly sharp. The man leaning casually against the rail at the side was her antagonist and rescuer of the day before. His bright blue eyes regarded her as she hesitated on the edge of the door.

'In you come. I was just looking for you. I'd like a word.' He stood upright and took a step towards her.

Alexis frowned. 'Sir. Is it one of the patients?' She withdrew her foot, preparing to go back down the corridor, and silently cursing the man. If she was to get a cuppa now was the time, and the minutes were ticking by, interruptions she didn't want. But she was too good a nurse to ignore a consultant's wants and needs on the ward.

'Did I say that?' Josh sniffed. 'I said I wanted a word with you.' Alexis stood poised on the threshold until the door threatened to close on her. 'For heavens sake, girl, come in here. I don't bite.' He extended a hand and gently grasped a wrist, drawing her inside the box of the lift and allowing the door to shut, before leaning over to press the ground floor button. Having apparently got his captive he didn't seem inclined to say anymore to her, however.

Alexis tried unobtrusively to remove his hand but he just smiled and took a firmer grip. 'Oh, no, I can see you slipping away.' She scowled at him, the hand wasn't oppressive and certainly not intended to hurt, but she didn't like being manhandled by men she didn't know.

He watched her face as the lift descended the three floors to the ground and then nodded. 'You need sugar. You're far too skinny and pale.'

'Well, re...' Alexis stopped herself. 'I am not in need of sugar... sir.' The last came out rather nastily.

'You're calling me, sir, again. And I know you didn't learn that in Kiwi land. Far too informal over there. The name is Josh, remember it.' He paused as the doors whooshed open. 'So you didn't do your training over there. Probably one of the London hospitals. They're a bit picky when it comes to protocol.' He released her wrist but walked closely beside her. 'We'll have a cup of coffee in the café. I'll get you an iced bun, it should do the trick.'

'I don't want an iced bun.' she scowled at his handsome face, then added a belated. 'Thank you.'

'You do you know, you just don't want to admit it.' His lips twitched. 'I'm going over there to get us coffee and cake. Wait here.' He indicated a small, wooden-topped, plastic table with four wooden chairs around it.

Alexis said, 'Woof woof.' under her breath and hesitated before sitting down. She did want tea or coffee or something; lunch was a distant memory and supper was still three hours away. But Josh whatever his name was, had a fine autocratic manner that set her teeth on edge a bit.

While she'd been watching him he'd approached the counter and given his order, made some comment that had the elderly lady who manned the café, smiling at him, and was headed back towards her. She'd wasted precious seconds watching, instead of wondering what he wanted and preparing her defence. Though just why she needed a defence she hadn't quite figured out yet. She just knew she did.

'Joyce says she'll bring it over in a minute.' He pulled out a chair. 'Now, I want you on my cardiac team. But April says I can't just poach you, because you probably want to stay with the babies. Well I understand that, until you can get some of your own, you can use others as a substitute, that's how some women are built.' He paused as a cup of coffee was set in front of him and a plate of cakes was placed in front of Alexis. The second cup of coffee swam into her vision and Josh nodded, 'Thanks a lot, Joyce. I appreciate it.'

Alexis meanwhile was opening and shutting her mouth, the scathing comment about male chauvinists hovering on her tongue waiting for the server of coffee to go away. She got in with her comment first. 'That's an appalling thing to say. I do not use other people's babies as substitutes. I enjoy my work, but I want more from my life than marriage and babies. I've never heard such old-fashioned ideas in my life!'

'Well, I'm glad you put marriage in there, I thought you were an old-fashioned girl, I'm glad to have it confirmed. It keeps you off my back. Nurses chasing me and not doing their work I can do without. Besides, it means I'll have you for a while, won't waste the training.'

Alexis shoved back her chair. 'Good God, you're Neolithic; I'm surprised you don't drag a club behind you and have trouble getting through doors the size of your head. Unless you have something pertinent to say about my work or patients, sir. I am going back to the ward.' She all but snarled at him as she prepared to stand up.

He touched her wrist. 'For God's sake, woman, stop being so touchy. I only meant you will work better if you are a career woman, not someone who is just looking for a free lunch.' He suddenly grinned, 'Speaking of which, drink your coffee and have something to eat.' He pushed the plate towards her.

'You are the most arrogant, impossible man I have ever met.'

'Can't have met many.' Josh grinned into her fuming face, 'What is your problem? I'm offering you a job.' The grin was turning to exasperation.

Alexis shook her head; she didn't know why he had this effect on her. She was normally cool headed. 'My apologies, sir. I must have misunderstood you; it sounded as if you were warning me off your person, while offering me that job.' The tone, saccharine sweet, made Josh wince slightly.

He looked at the oval face and the stormy eyes. 'Oops! That wasn't my intention at all.' He shook his head in his turn. 'Look, let's start again. I thought your handling of the minor emergency with the Jones baby showed promise, I would like you to come and work for me.' He paused, 'If you would also like to transfer to cardiac.'

Alexis was already shaking her head at him. He didn't give her time to explain.

'Why not, it's just as fascinating as babies, more so, at least the patients can tell you what's wrong, and they have lived, they have stories to tell. Unless you've got a boyfriend and are waiting to have your own.' He could hear the annoyance in his own voice and tried to quell it. The hazel eyes looked sad now.

'They aren't taking any more staff on, sir.' She watched the scowl forming on his face. 'I'm agency. Anyway I can't accept a permanent job in the hospital, even if there was a job going. I'll be leaving the area in the next three weeks anyway. Peter needs me, and Mary needs a break.'

'Oh.' He fell silent, just staring at her. There was a Peter, who needed her. Suddenly that mattered much more than the fact that he couldn't poach her from the Mother and Baby Ward.

Alexis watched him as he stared into his cup of coffee. She picked up her own cup and began to drink the cooling brew. She tried to get a surreptitious look at her watch, but her cardigan was covering the face of the fob. She needed to get back on the ward;

her break must be nearly up.

'Stop looking at your watch, I'll take you back and explain to Gill.' He had a way of noticing when you least expected it, she thought. 'Eat something. I wasn't wrong about you needing sugar. You nurses either comfort eat, or starve yourselves to pay the rent. Unless you're on some tom-fool diet?' He paused, the question delicately balanced between inquiry about her financial state or worries for her figure.

Alexis took an iced finger and took a healthy bite just to prove him wrong, chewing and swallowing before answering him, 'My figure is no-one's concern but mine, sir. And nor are my finances.'

'I'm pleased to hear it, and if you call me sir, one more time I shall...I shall kiss you in this very public hall and embarrass us both. Do I make myself clear?'

Alexis about to say, 'Yes, sir,' swallowed the thought and took another bite of iced bun to keep the ill advised words from leaking out.

'Good.' He nodded at her. 'Now I might be able to swing something if you wanted a permanent job here. Do you?' He waited impatiently for her eyebrows to lower from their astonished position, 'I have a little influence with the board.'

This time it was Alexis who said nothing more than, 'Oh!' and sat still staring at her hands. A permanent job, in cardiac, her dream job. But so far from Mother Mary, from the foster home, the safety of caring for the children who came and went and needed her. From little Peter, whose mixed race mother had rejected him, from Carl suffering from the affects of foetal alcohol syndrome, from Eva whose only fault was that she wasn't a pretty child. She had promised Mother Mary that she would come back after she had some experience under her belt.

She shook her head at her own thoughts and Josh, not privy to them, growled next to her. What was she thinking about, rejecting a plum job and jobs so scarce? It had become important to him to get this young woman for his team. He wasn't, yet, quite sure why.

Mother Mary would tell her to go for it, that she could manage fine, as she always did, that she wasn't going to take anymore foster children after this, but she always did. She'd only ever adopted three and Alexis was one of the three. The boys had made good careers, they returned at frequent intervals but they couldn't help in the way she could.

She looked at Josh. 'I'm sorry, I appreciate the offer but I have to get back.' She wondered, as did Josh, whether she meant back to the ward or back to her Peter. She stood up, 'Thank you for my coffee.'

Josh who had stood up as she rose, nodded, 'I'll let Gill know that I detained you.' He watched her walk away towards the bank of lifts and pulled out his mobile.

Chapter 3.

COMING OFF DUTY AT ten at night, Alexis was greeted by rain and more rain. It dripped from the end of her nose and she gave a swipe at it with a mitten clad hand. 'I hate British summers!' She spoke to herself as she made her way across the car park and out through the heavy wrought iron gates onto the pavement outside the redbrick Victorian area of the hospital. 'And summers in Cumbria are worse than summers in Britain.

'That, Alexis, is a contradiction, or possibly a gerund. My grammar never was very good. It was the despair of my tutors.' Alexis visibly jumped as the man at the gate spoke to her.

Josh stopped leaning against the gatepost and took her arm. 'I imagine you are planning on walking through the park and along the riverside, which let me tell you, is not a safe thing to do, even in Carlisle.'

Alexis looked up at him through a veil of wet hair and raindrops. 'Good evening, s...' she hastily changed it to 'Mr Blevins.'

'Ah! Been asking questions about me have you?'

Alexis shook her head. 'Gill told me that Mr Blevins had rung to explain why I was a few minutes late back from my break, ergo you are Mr Blevins.'

'Oh, now that is disappointing. I thought you might have made a few inquiries and changed your mind about the job. Indeed I was hoping, now you've had time to think about it, you would see some sense and decide to join us. That's why I met you at the gates. I've just finished myself.'

She sighed. 'I'm sorry I can't do that.' They walked in silence for a few paces along the roadway, 'How did you know I was a New Zealander?' Alexis glanced up and away checking to see how annoyed he was and hoping to change the subject.

'I've never heard any other group of people describe themselves as being 'right as a box of fluffies'.' I did a one year locum down there just after I qualified. Lovely people.'

For the first time, Josh saw her beautiful smile. 'Where did you work, Josh?'

His heart, a well regulated organ as befitted a cardiac surgeon, gave a quick leap. 'Bay of Plenty. Lively volcanoes and the odd earthquake aside, its gorgeous country; almost as pretty as mine. I enjoyed my time there enormously. Do you know the area?'

Alexis shook her head. 'We never left the South Island until mum and I came back.'

Josh would have liked to ask why they had returned to Britain, but didn't. He told himself it was none of his business, which it wasn't, that he didn't need to know her background to employ her, which he didn't, yet he could still feel the questions forming a queue on his tongue. He shook the rain off his face and stopped walking.

Alexis had perforce to stop too. She looked at him.

'Can I give you a lift home, Alexis?'

'I only live a little way from the park, Mr Blevins.'

'Now don't go all formal on me again.' He grinned, water dripping from his rain-darkened hair. 'I'm only offering you a lift.' He indicated his Cherokee parked on the roadside and held the door invitingly open for her.

Alexis hesitated, and then decided that this odd consultant was surely to be trusted. She swung herself up into the high seat of the four-by-four, and then gave a yelp as something soft squeaked under her bottom. She hastily raised herself and pulled a floppy, cloth doll out from underneath her, holding it up to reveal the glory of yellow hair and a gingham dress with long pink legs and painted-on black shoes.

Josh was just climbing into the driver's seat. He looked across at her in the fading light as she frankly giggled at him. 'I thought I'd sat on a cat or something.'

'Ah! I'd forgotten where I put that.' Josh took the doll and set it on the back seat. 'Emma's reward.'

'Emma?'

Josh ignored the question for one of his own. 'You live in those flats along near the riverside don't you? At least that's where you set off for yesterday.'

Alexis cast a look at the doll lolling on the back seat. Apparently she wasn't going to get an answer. Maybe Emma was his daughter and a daughter argued a wife. Maybe that's why he wanted to 'keep her off his back.' She realised he was waiting for an answer. 'Er, yes, that's right.'

She subsided into the seat as he swung the car in a neat u-turn and set off, up the road. Alexis's mind was busy adding two and two and coming up with five. If he had a wife he shouldn't have kissed her, and that meant he wasn't to be trusted that much. She scowled at the windscreen, her eyes tracking the repetitious movement of the wipers. Maybe all that talk of keeping women at bay was a way of testing them out to see who was available. She frowned some more. He'd threatened to kiss her in the café too.

Josh cast a glance at his now very silent, passenger, wondering just what she was thinking. He didn't talk about Emma. Not because he was ashamed of her, but because he didn't talk about his private life at the hospital. He'd deliberately parked a small stroll away from the gates so that the gossip mill might not see. He told himself he was just trying to get a good nurse for his team, and then sniffed at the rain still running down his face. Actually he wasn't quite sure what his motives were with regard to Alexis, but he didn't want to advertise them, he was very sure of that.

She came out of her reverie to discover he was driving slowly along the line of old semis that had been divided into student accommodation for the nursing staff of the hospital some years before. He knew this because he'd inherited them from his father, and then gifted them to the hospital for the nurses, when nursing hostels no longer became popular or practical.

'What number?'

'Five.'

He pulled up neatly at the curb and began to get out.

Alexis was too quick for him. 'Thank you for the lift, sir.' She stepped back from the door and slammed it shut.

Josh, undoing his seatbelt, started to speak, 'Now wait just...' He stopped as his beeper sounded in the silence of the evening. 'Damn. We haven't done, young lady.' He refastened the belt, 'Duty calls.' He raised a hand in farewell and turned the big four-by-four, driving off in a fine spray of water. Alexis watched the red tail lights disappearing round the end of the street and then sighed deeply.

'Well, that was interesting, Alexis, now get you body out of the rain and your mind out of the gutter.' She couldn't decide who she was more angry with, Josh for offering her things just that bit out of her reach like Tantalus on a spree, or herself for allowing her mind to stray just a tiny bit towards thoughts of what it would be like to have a second kiss.

JOSH MEANWHILE WAS HEADING back to the hospital, 'Why

did I choose medicine? I could lead a life of leisure. I could go and live on the family estate.' He muttered to himself as he pulled up in the courtyard around the back of the hospital. With a slight squeal of his brakes on the wet surface, and dismissing Alexis from his mind, he strode into the hospital, talking on his phone.

'OK, I'm on the premises; I'll be there in a couple of minutes. Get a drip up, normal saline over four hours to start with, administer aspirin if possible, and do an ECG as soon as you get him into his bed.' He kept walking, headed up to the cardiac ward and Andrew Hardy.

They'd got him bagged with a rebreather, oxygen running a 6 millilitres through the mask. He was on the floor of the toilets in the four bed ward. The night charge nurse was busy replacing the cannula in his right arm; another nurse was just wheeling up his bed so that they could do a direct transfer from the floor to the bed.

'How did he come to be out of bed?' Josh raised an eyebrow.

Andrew Hardy spoke through the muffling plastic of the mask, 'Wanted number two's.' He puffed the words out.

'And what did I tell you before I left this afternoon?' He shook his head gently at his patient. 'Here's another fine mess you've got yourself in. Let's get you back into bed, how's the pain on a scale of 10?'

'About 7, Doc.'

Josh waited while three nurses and the night

charge-nurse lifted and settled him, and then wheeled the bed back to its position against the wall. 'Show me where?'

Andrew Hardy, lifted his right arm and pointed to his left arm, then carried the fingers onwards and upwards. 'Hurts my teeth, so it can't be me ticker, can it?'

'I'm afraid it can, Mr Hardy. At least you're in the right place if you're determined to have a heart attack.' Josh pulled a portable trolley over, fixing oximeter and BP cuff on the right arm. He flicked a stethoscope from the top of the trolley and laid the cup over the hairy chest exposed on the bed.

'Let's have 5ml of morph and max drawn up to take away the pain, staff.' He looked at the man on the bed, 'It'll help the pain and make you a bit sleepy, Andrew. OK?' Josh might have asked, but the nurse was busy checking the vial of pain relief with another nurse even as he spoke, laying the syringe ready in a dish with some normal saline. I'll just get the ECG done so we can see exactly what is going on in there before we do that, if you don't mind, staff.'

The ECG machine was already being wheeled into the room. Josh stood back and watched as his team did the various tests carefully, but rapidly, then administered the pain relief. He spoke quietly to the Charge, 'I think I might shift him to ICU, Bill, if we can find a bed. I don't think we've seen the last of this.

Bill Sharpe nodded. 'I'll ring through, Josh.'

Josh nodded back in acknowledgement and then took the ECG that had just been handed to him.

'He's in A Fib, let's give some Digoxin and Calcium Gluconate as well, it looks like a STEMI from the readout.' He turned to one of the nurses, 'Streptokinase, usual dose and a glycoprotein, let's get him back on an even keel for the present and reduce the risk of clots, then transfer as soon as Bill gets back to you. I don't want to operate when I'm so tired, but...' Josh tailed away. 'Let's try and get him stabilised until tomorrow.'

Bill appeared next to him. 'All fixed Josh. They're expecting him upstairs and I've booked him in for CABG first thing, if he signs the form.'

'Good, Let's hope those skinny legs have got some decent veins in them, Bill.' Josh nodded at him and then watched as Andrew Hardy was wheeled away to the ICU. His theatre sister would not be happy to find she'd got a coronary artery bypass graft fixed for first thing when she'd got all her lists nicely organised, but it couldn't be helped.

ALEXIS WAS TALKING ABOUT helping. Mary thought differently however. 'It sounds to me like the ideal job, Alexis. Why don't you want to take it?'

'Because, it's a long way from home and I want to help you and the other children. I promised you.'

Mary nodded. 'I hear what you say, love, but are you sure that's the only reason?' The question was proffered gently but Mary gave her, 'The Look', perfected over years of dealing with difficult children. 'You need to think about your motives, Alexis.' Mary always made the children she rescued and nurtured think about why they did things.

Alexis frowned at the screen; she offered a half smile, 'We should have done this over the telephone then you couldn't get to me.'

'Ah ha, so you do have other reasons, love.'

Alexis wrinkled her nose. 'I don't know, maybe, it's just I thought if I rang you, you would reassure me that I'm doing the right thing, and now I'm all confused again.'

'You, Alexis Bowen, have never been confused, you duck and dodge issues, you hide from the truth at times, but you aren't confused.' Mary shook her head at her adopted daughter.

'OK,' Alexis nodded, accepting the description of her character. 'I'm going to take the weekend off. I'll see you tomorrow night. I'm late shift so I'll be very late, Mother Mary. I will think, but a promise is a promise.'

'Yes, love. I know, always keep your promises and threats, that's what I taught you, but I don't expect you to keep promises you gave when you where only a bairn.'

'I've renewed it since I was an adult!' Alexis looked indignantly at the screen.

'Aye, yes.' Mary lapsed into her native Yorkshire, 'Happen you have, but you aren't going to hide here, my lamb.'

'Mother Mary!' Alexis stopped as the screen face smiled softly at her and held up a finger. 'Alright,

I'll talk to you tomorrow.'

'Love you, Lexy. Tomorrow it is. I'll kill the fatted calf.' Mary gave a brief wave and the screen went blank.

Alexis closed the lid of her laptop and sat back in the comfortable easy chair. The machine rested on her legs, still warm from the conversation. 'I'm not hiding am I?' She addressed the empty air. 'I don't think I am.' She stood up, setting the machine on the small coffee table, and went into the kitchenette to make a last drink before bedtime.

THE MORNING DIDN'T BRING any wiser council. Alexis, busy packing a weekend bag and then moving on to emptying the small fridge of things that might go off over the weekend, sighed. She almost wished she could be packing up and going home for good. She sat back on her heels, holding the cloth she'd been wiping the bottom of fridge with, and looked blankly at the near empty interior. 'Maybe I am running away.'

She rubbed her nose with a wet hand. Then shoved her head further inside the machine to reach the back of the salad draw. She addressed a pat of butter. 'Botheration. I was getting along fine; it's all that consultant's fault.' Then she shook her head and gave a final swipe to the plastic before dropping the cloth with a sploosh into a bowl of water next to her.

'I will not hide, I will not run away. I will clean up my own mess.' She nodded to herself as she picked up the bowl and turned to empty the contents into the sink. She was just putting the cloth over the taps when the doorbell rang. 'Now what?' She glanced at her watch, 'One 'o'clock.' It better hadn't be double glazing or someone offering to save her. She hadn't got time either to argue or explain her position regarding either need.

The door opened to reveal Josh on the doorstep resplendent in jeans and a cashmere sweater she itch to run her hand over however Alexis stood with the door in that hand, and an equally wooden expression on her face.

Josh smiled, his blue eyes crinkled in what was becoming an all too familiar way, and his lips lifted. 'Can I come in?'

Alexis regarded him for a moment more. 'You can, but you may not, Mr Blevins.'

Josh regarded her, the smile retreating in the face of such non-encouragement. 'I was passing; I wondered if you might like lunch before work?'

'No, thank you.' Icicles formed around the words.

Josh pretended to shiver, 'Chilly around here.' He shrugged, 'All I'm offering is lunch. I won't pressure you to take the job, but I meant it, I can get you onto my team.' He'd spent an urgent, and not entirely fraught-free half hour, contacting one of the members of the board, arguing his case; it now looked as though it had been a waste of time and effort.

Alexis shook her head.

Josh waited for her to say something, and in the meantime looked at what he could see of her small flat. 'Hey! I really mean it. I won't pressure you; you don't have to move out.' He looked horrified as he continued to stare at the overnight suitcase resting in the hall.

Alexis looked at him in astonishment, and then looked in the direction his eyes seemed to be fixed. For the first time she relaxed into a tiny smile. 'I'm going away for the weekend.' Now why had she told him that? He didn't need to know her plans.

'Phew!' He pretended to flick sweat from his brow. 'You'll be back then?'

Alexis nodded. 'Sunday afternoon.'

Josh wasn't sure what was going wrong with his heart, it was going up and down like a pea in a lift. Bouncing and rolling around in his chest. In fact he wasn't quite sure what was wrong with him that kept him fixed on this doorstep, when it was quite obvious she was wishing him anywhere but there.

'Look, Alexis,' He offered a tentative smile; 'It has to be Alexis, I don't know your second name. Can we start again?' He held out his hand, 'Hi, I'm Josh Blevins, I work at the hospital.'

Alexis ignored the hand. 'I am aware of your position in the hospital, Mr Blevins, and I don't mix with the upper echelons of the hospital hierarchy. I don't mix with married men either. It only leads to trouble.'

Josh was becoming tired of the brush-off he was getting. He wasn't used to it; his smile had got him into, and out of, trouble, all his life. Girls usually wanted to be with him. He frowned. His next comment wasn't in English. It also wasn't very polite. *Pentwp, rhodi'r ffidil yn y tô.* He turned and walked away, heading down the three steps that led to the garden path and gate.

Alexis was left staring at the empty doorway and listening to the rapid retreat of hand-made shoes on the stones of the path. 'Hmm, that went well, so much for not hiding and not running away, Lexy.' She shut the door and went back to getting ready for her shift.

JOSH MEANWHILE WAS MUTTERING to himself, 'What does she mean married men, I'm not married. I wonder who's been telling tales, and inaccurate ones at that.' He got into his car and revved the engine quite unnecessarily to relieve his temper, before driving off to the hospital, gravel spitting behind the turning wheels. He would go and see if Andrew Hardy had come out of post op. He should have done that instead of trying to make her see sense. He didn't assign a name to her, he knew who he meant and he didn't understand why he was so set on seeing more of her. He had enough skilled people on his team.

He strode into the ICU and walked over to the bedside. Mr Hardy was connected to more tubes than the London Underground. Saline dripped remorselessly into one arm, a drain came out of his chest into a bag which was attached to the side of the bed. A catheter snaked down and drained into a bag of urine on the other side of the bed. A BP cuff was just finishing its routine check of his blood pressure and another machine was supplying him with a steady dose of pain relief.

'I take it he's come round, Staff?'

The Staff Nurse gave him an odd look, 'He's down here, Josh, post-op would have kept him otherwise.'

'Stable?' The question came out with something of a bark.

'Yes, he's doing nicely now. Another forty-eight hours and we can send him back to Cardiac.'

'I'll decide when he goes back.'

The Staff Nurse looked at him with such astonishment that Josh swallowed his comment and shook his head. 'Sorry, lot on my mind. You're quite right, you have more than enough experience to judge when he's ready to go.' He spun on his heel and left the bedside and the room. The Staff Nurse watched him go and then looked at her friend, 'What was that all about? He usually stands back and gives us the credit for things.'

'Is Mr Hardy not well?'

'He's doing great, Josh did a lovely job on the graft, beautiful stitching on the leg too.'

They looked at each other and shrugged. 'Oh well, back to work.'

Josh, meantime, was walking rapidly towards his office; he was in a foul temper, such an unusual state of affairs that he thought he'd better hide in his office until he calmed down. He didn't get the chance.

His pager went off as he had a hand on the doorknob, '*Chch!*' He glanced at the readout and turned, going up to the post-op ward.

'Sister Jenkins?'

'Threadgold, sir. His blood pressure is dropping. I think he must have a bleeder.'

Josh nodded, going over to his final patient of the morning. He'd performed a triple bypass on the elderly man. It had been a struggle finding veins good enough in the legs; he'd had to cut far deeper than he wanted to. He examined the reddened bindings. 'Yeah, you're right, let's get him prepped and back into surgery. I must have been careless.'

'I very much doubt that, sir.' Sister Jenkins was nearing retirement, very professional and used to all sorts of consultants. She thought Josh was one of the best, unfailingly polite to both staff and patients alike, so she was somewhat shocked to hear him swear again under his breath. It might have been in Welsh, but she still knew what it meant.

'*Uffern Dân.*' Josh heard the intake of breath and looked sheepishly at her. 'Sorry, Meg, I forgot you spoke Welsh. I can usually get away with it.'

'Well, we're not much good at swearing as a rule, but we can blaspheme with the best of them can't we? Off you go and get scrubbed; I'll have him wheeled in, in ten minutes.' She offered a forgiving smile. 'I shouldn't think you've been careless at all, sir.'

Josh pushed his frustration and annoyance to

the back of his mind and went into the operating theatre, where he was kept busy, re-opening and finding, then stitching up, the small artery that was leaking into the surrounding tissue and out of Mr Threadgold's leg.

He didn't have any time to dwell on the odd behaviour, or wrong information that Alexis appeared to possess, until nearly eight that night. An MI had been admitted, swiftly followed by one of his private patient's whose Atrial valve was leaking and required some painstaking work to ensure the woman had a future.

By that time he'd been on his feet for over fourteen hours, and despite his urgent desire to get things sorted out he was just too tired. He went home and sat brooding until he fell asleep before the gas fire and had to take himself, stiff and rumpled, to his bed at midnight.

Chapter 4.

ALEXIS WAS ALSO A bit stiff at midnight. After her shift she'd driven the fifty odd miles from Carlisle to Whitehaven in her blue Ford Focus. Driving in the Lake District was one of her delights. She revelled in the scenery, but not much of that could be seen at ten at night. Night driving required more concentration than she had thought after eight hours on the ward.

Mary was on the lookout for her even so, and had her into the house and a comfortable chair hardly before she'd taken her coat off. Young Peter, apparently as bright as a button, was ensconced on her knee playing with her plait, while Mary made the tea. She came through bearing two mugs on a tray. 'Good journey?'

'Quiet, not many people stupid enough to be on the roads at this time of night.'

Mary half grinned at her, the side of her mouth lifting. 'You could have come tomorrow morning, love.'

She got a shake of the head. 'I wanted two full days of your company, mother Mary.'

'Do you want to talk now?'

'No. I'm just glad to be home. It's been a funny sort of week.' She grinned, 'I think I've been sworn at.'

'Think? I generally know fine when folks swear at me.'

'Who would dare swear at you, mother?'

'Not many. But the odd doctor has, when I won't give up on my babies.'

'Now that I can believe!' Alexis leaned forward and took a sip of tea, whilst settling Peter who was now sucking his thumb and resting against her. His chocolate brown eyes starting to droop. 'Another few minutes and he'll be asleep.' Alexis looked down on the riot of brown curls on the two-year-old's head. 'He looks well.'

Mary Down nodded. 'Yes, it was cruel, the way his mother treated him, fancy starving a little mite just because his skin's too dark for her family's taste. He's their grandchild, their daughter conceived him, if he'd been a blue eyed blond like his ma there wouldn't have been any problems. But no, to leave him in his cot like that...' Mary shook her head, 'he's such a darling too.'

'You aren't thinking of...' Alexis tailed away as she caught the guilty look on Mary's face. 'Mother Mary, what have you done?'

'Nothing yet.' She grinned, 'I can't, I haven't had him long enough, but I'm only forty; I can adopt if I want to.' It was said a shade defiantly. 'The only trouble is they keep talking about "placing within his own culture", and I ask you, what when it gets down to it, is that? He's as much white as Caribbean.'

Alexis grinned. 'So just how far have you got?'

'Not far, if we can find out where his other grandparents are, he might have a home with them instead.'

'And you'll be sad?'

Mary shook her head. 'No, I love him, but I want what he needs best, and if he has a family who want him, then I'll let him go to them.'

'You took me.'

'You had no-one. And you were damaged, darling, and I loved you.'

Alexis smiled over the now sleeping child. 'Amen to that.'

'Come on, love, time that young man was abed, and you too, you're dropping before my eyes. I'll come and tuck you in.' Mary gave a chuckle at the look on her adopted daughter's face. 'Not too old for a goodnight kiss are you?'

'Never from you, Mother.' Alexis looked at the lined face and the grey hair of the woman in front of her. Her foster mother was pretty but she was beautiful when she smiled as she did now.

True to her word Mary Down, after a quick knock, came into the bedroom ten minutes later and, proffering a hot water bottle, leaned over and kissed Alexis on the brow. 'We'll talk tomorrow, love.'

Alexis nodded and snuggled down. She should have settled down and been asleep in minutes, but she wasn't. She lay, warm bottle hugged against her body more for comfort than warmth, thinking about the encounter with Josh Blevins earlier that day.

She could picture the blue eyes and hear the exasperation in his voice. She wondered what he'd said and what language he'd said it in. His daughter would be pretty if she had his eyes. She started to scowl as she thought about what kind of wife he would have. She'd lay odds his wife wouldn't be 'damaged'. Unless it was by his infidelity.

Her hands moved down the bed and rubbed the top of her thighs where the thin, white lines of old scars bore testimony to the damage. She could understand that kind of emotional betrayal very easily. She had dealt with it by self-inflicted pain, the scars a testimony to her need to find some relief from the loss of both parents and the fear of being alone; for someone to listen and understand. Thank God Mother Mary had done just that. Eventually she fell asleep to dream of a brown-eyed baby crying piteously in a room with no door. She was glad to wake up.

So was Josh. Saturdays he took his daughter to the baths. She couldn't swim, but she loved getting into the water with her wings on and floating in his arms. She would splash and chuckle and no matter how hard his week had been she never failed to put a smile on his face.

Today was different though, he could see that as soon as he woke. No imp of mischief was sitting on his chest as usual. He climbed out of bed, glanced at the clock, and frowned. Normally she was awake by six-thirty and now it was nearly an hour later.

He pulled on his jeans and, still tugging his polo t-shirt down over his chest, went in search of his daughter. 'Maria.' He strode into Emma's bedroom. His daughter was still asleep; her lips slightly blue, her breathing a bit shallow.

Maria was busy in the corner, she was adjusting a portable oxygen cylinder and fitting a tube and mask onto it. 'I thought she sleeping well. She look alright at seven. But when I check just now I notice how blue she going.'

'Alright, Maria, let's get her hooked up and then I'll examine her. She probably just has a bit of a cold; she was breathless yesterday morning. How was she for the rest of the day?'

'She had her inhalers four times, but she seem OK, Dottore.'

Josh nodded, watching as she expertly fitted the mask. Emma wasn't objecting, which she sometimes did; she wasn't actually stirring at all. 'I'll just get my bag; six litres and get her propped up a bit.'

He returned with his medical bag and a stethoscope in his hand. His daughter opened her eyes as he undid the buttons of her pyjama top. 'Hello, daddy.'

'Hello, my Emma, daddy needs to listen to your chest. If you're good you can have your new dolly in bed with you.'

'Dolly?' She gave a very tired smile.

'Yes, 'Dolly'. She's called;' he searched his mind for distractions while the black clouds of worry bumped against the professional clouds of understanding. 'Lexy. I know a nurse called Lexy, isn't that a funny name? She's very pretty and she's got long blonde hair too' His daughter nodded and watched him as he placed the bell of the stethoscope on her chest, listening first to her upper lungs, then her heart. 'Lean forward for me, darling.'

He glanced at Maria, who stepped forward and held the child as he listened to the lower lobes at the back of the thin chest. 'Now let's take your temp, OK. He showed the small instrument that went into her ear. 'You've had that done before haven't you? You know it doesn't hurt.'

Emma nodded and held still while he inserted and waited for the beep. Josh glanced at the read-out. 'You aren't very well, darling, no swimming today, I'm sorry, but I promise to sit with you and read you a story this morning after you've had a wash and eaten some breakfast.'

'Don't want any.' A small mutinous lip trembled and the brown eyes filled with tears, 'Want to go swimmin.' The mask was pulled half off and got tangled in the pudgy fingers.

Josh nodded. 'I know, I like going swimming with you too.' He took the mask, untangled it and replaced it on her face. 'But your poor chest isn't very well. I'm going to give you some medicine too.' He motioned to Maria. 'Turn her over I'll give it into her bottom.' Emma wasn't very happy about that and squirmed and cried, but she rapidly exhausted her store of energy. And lay back against the pillows after he'd quickly inserted the paracetamol and Maria had redressed her.

'Now I'm going to get dolly, but she can only stay in the bed if you keep the mask on.' He looked at Maria. 'I'm going to get the pharmacy to make up some Amoxicillin. Her chest is very congested.' He offered a half smile. 'She'll be a handful. If you can give her a bit of a wash and I'll see what I can do about breakfast.'

He returned minutes later with the cloth doll. His daughter was apparently asleep again but her colour was better. He could hear sounds of Maria in the adjoining bathroom running water and he dropped the doll on the bed and retreated. He would go and arrange something for them both to eat while battle commenced in the bedroom.

Joan, the housekeeper, was already awake and busy in the kitchen. She had a pan on the stove and toasted fingers keeping warm under the grill. 'Poor wee lamb, see if you can get her to eat some egg and soldiers. I've found her favourite egg-cup.'

Josh merely smiled; Joan seemed to know what was going on in his house long before he did, 'I'm bribing her with story time. She isn't going to like the medicine.'

'Well, nor did you, Josh. If she won't take it from you, you can always bring up the reserves.' She pointed at her chest.

He grinned; it lit his eyes for a few seconds.

'She's going to be a right pain when she's over the worst.'

'Aren't they all?' But Joan saw the same fear in his eyes. Little Emma hadn't got the capital to fight off a major infection and they both knew it.

ALEXIS WAS ALSO EATING eggs and soldiers. Or rather say, she was trying to. Peter was sitting in his high chair, but so near that he kept stealing fingers of toast and stuffing them in his mouth even as he giggled at her. 'Peter, that's naughty.' Mary shook her head at him as she turned around from the stove in the comfortable kitchen and brought a brown teapot to the laden table.

He grinned around his new teeth and wiped his fingers through his hair. Mary just sighed and gave him a slice of toast for himself.

'It never tastes as good as the stolen stuff. Why do you think that is?' Alexis moved her own meal out of range, even while she offered bread to Carl. Carl was nearly four but his head flopped a bit and he needed help to eat properly. Sometimes you even won a smile from him, but it was a rare event for strangers. She looked at Mary even as she fed the child. 'Have we heard...?'

'His mother wants him back. And the social say she can have him. The poor little soul's like a pin-pong ball. She cleans up her act then falls off the wagon and back he comes to me, the trouble is she genuinely loves him. And that counts in the long run, Lexy.'

Cardiac Arrest

'When does he go?'

'End of the week. You'll like seeing mummy again won't you, Carl?' Mary dropped a kiss on the tousled blond curls, and big green eyes looked at her before a gappy smile lit his face. Mary won smiles easily from Carl. 'They are making his granny guardian, and he stays with mum only if mum stays with her mother. This is her last chance.'

A small girl came into the kitchen trailing one shoe and a battered teddy. 'Mum, mum, there's a car...Oh, Lexy, how lovely.' Eva raised a face which would have been handsome on a Rear Admiral, but on a small child was all teeth and nose. 'When did you come? Are you staying? Can we go shopping together again?' The questions arrived as if fired from a gun. The face might have been ugly but the smile was beautiful on the eight-year-old's face. Eva came and leaned against Alexis's shorts-clad leg confident of her welcome and unconscious of a face which would cause her enormous grief in the years to come.

'Let Lexy finish her breakfast, and you get yours, pet.'

Eva slid onto the next seat and smiled, 'Can I have eggs and soldiers too?'

'Course you can. Help Carl for a minute while I get it ready.'

Alexis sat back with her mug of coffee and watched as Eva held the young boy's head and fed him egg from a specially shaped spoon. 'There you go, Carl, eat it all up like a good boy.'

She swapped a spoon for a tippy mug, and wrapped Carl's hands around the two handles, holding his head up so that he could feed himself. Alexis and Mary exchanged a glance; here was a natural 'mother', but given the child's lack of attributes it was unlikely she would become one.

When the breakfast was over and the daily tasks of washing up and bed-making completed, Mary decreed that the swings was to be the next stop. 'We might get a chance to talk while Eva gets rid of some energy and Peter goes on the swings, otherwise you'll have to save it until bedtime, love.' Mary shrugged even as she smiled.

'I know, Mother, that was always the way.'

As it turned out Eva found a friend at the playground, a girl of her own age who was in a wheelchair. She rushed off to help and Mary sat on one of the benches next to the swings with a slight sigh. Alexis picked up Carl, then Peter, and strapped them into seats and began to gently push them alternately getting giggles from Peter and a smile from Carl for her pains.

Mary admired the slim figure of her daughter in the shorts and t-shirt. 'It must be nearly summer- you're showing off your figure.' She herself had still got a jumper on and was glad of it; the wind off the sea, some distance away, was a bit chilly for her liking. Mary spoke as she watched them. 'So what's the problem, Lexy?'

'I told you, I feel I should come home and lend a hand. This job, it sounds good, but I'm not sure about the consultant who's offering it. He seemed nice enough, but then first he insulted me and then he waited for me after shift. I'm a bit wary of him.'

'Is he nice, what does he look like?'

'Mother!' A note of exasperation sounded.

'If I'm your mother I'm entitled to ask those questions.' Mary sniffed, 'So...'

Alexis frowned. 'He's got blue, blue eyes, dark hair, a lovely smile.' She paused; she hadn't realised she'd taken that much notice. 'I think he's got money, but then most consultants have, he wears one of those signet rings on his little finger. Nice suits. He wears nice suits on the ward, some of the younger doctors, you can hardly tell them from the porters, and they look so scruffy.'

'Hmm, and?'

'What do you mean 'and'?'

'Well, why don't you want the job?'

'He might be married?'

'What's that got to do with the job?'

Alexis shook her head, her braid swinging at her back. 'I got the feeling he was coming on to me.'

'So, if he's married, tell him no.'

'But I couldn't work with someone who was...well you know.'

Mary nodded. 'Fine, I agree, it would make life difficult and there are other jobs. But wouldn't it be better to find out first?' She sniffed again.

Alexis wrinkled her nose, 'Yes, one of these

two needs a nappy change. See, you have got a lot on your plate with this lot, too much to manage on your own.' She avoided her foster mother's eye as she avoided answering the question. For some reason she wasn't going to examine, she didn't want to get involved, and any excuse was better than none.

Mary was speaking and Alexis only caught the tail end of the sentence. 'I'll only have two by the end of the week, and Eva is at school most of the day.'

'But you're thinking of taking on Peter full time.' She gave the little boy a quick push and heard his chuckle. 'It's not been as easy since Ralf…'

'No, I miss my husband every day.' Mary shook her head. 'You need to live your life, love. I didn't bring you up and spend all that energy on you, for you to be under my feet now.'

Alexis, frankly grinned. 'Cheek! Under your feet indeed! Who's the one standing here pushing?'

Mary's lips twitched. 'I love you, Lexy, you know that, but you have to make a life of your own.' She paused, 'You're hiding, love, don't you think I know the signs by now. We all have to get hurt, to feel pain, to experience life, Alexis.'

Mary moved, standing and beginning to gently push Carl. 'I know you're afraid, Alexis, but you faced the challenge of training, away from home. You managed to move out, now I want you to form relationships outside the safety of my house. Do you understand, Alexis?

'I feared for you when Ralf died. I wondered if

you might resort to old habits. But you didn't. You aren't hiding the scars; you used to do that, now you ignore them.' She laid a work roughened hand on Alexis's arm for a minute. 'I was proud of you then. Make me more proud, love.'

Alexis bit her lip, but the reply she might have made stayed on her tongue as Eva came over holding the hand of a strange woman. 'Mum, this is Elizabeth and her little girl, Susan, she has got spiny biffs,' Eva stumbled over the words, 'and they say I can come to tea this afternoon and they only live in the next street. Can I go, please?'

Alexis stepped back and lifted the two boys one by one out of their seats and into the double buggy, strapping them in. Mary moved aside slightly to explain that, while Susan and her mother were more than welcome to visit and have tea with Eva, Eva, because she was in a foster home couldn't go to other houses without some checks being made about those homes.

Alexis sighed. It wasn't easy being fostered, and the law made it more difficult. You were, 'different', little things that made the other children look at you. Not being able to have friends to tea or for sleepovers was just the tip of the iceberg. While Alexis understood, as an adult, the precautions set in place; it made the already vulnerable even more so.

Mary hated the look of disappointment on Eva's face but the law was strict. Elizabeth Hutchins nodded. 'Would you like to see where Eva lives, Susan?'

Susan beamed and nodded vigorously, from her safety of her wheelchair. 'Oh yes.' She was a pretty child and the contrast could have been cruel but the smiles of both children's faces were the same a beam of acceptance of each other.

'Then we'll come to you for tea today and next time you can come to us.' She and Mary exchanged a look.

'I'll set things up if you would like that. I'll explain all about the police checks and social workers this afternoon. It can be a bit daunting.' Mary paused, watching the other woman's face, expecting to see rejection, but she got a nod.

'That would be good. About fourish?'

TEA TIME SAW EMMA sitting up in bed, the second dose of antibiotic beginning to do some work in her system and the Panadol reducing her temperature. She was, however, still far from well, and it was taking the combined efforts of three adults to keep her entertained and in bed.

The new doll was a success, having the place of honour next to her on the pillow and being offered biscuits and kisses in equal proportions. Josh had read several stories over the morning and Joan had taken over in the afternoon, dressing dolly in a few clothes from other dolls while he dealt with the post and several phone calls. Emma was now getting tired and fretful, however. Her latest request was to meet the real Lexy. This was a circumstance that Josh had not foreseen. In fact he hadn't thought that Emma had taken in that much of the conversation.

'I can't do that, darling. She's probably at work. Looking after poorly children.' He frowned to himself, no, not that, she was away, he remembered now. He shook his head at his daughter.

'M poorly, Daddy, she can cum 'n look after me.' Emma rubbed her eyes and frowned at her father sitting next to her in the low rocking chair.

'I can't get her today, darling, besides you have Joan and Maria and me to look after you.'

'Want, Lexy.'

Josh shook his head and pulled her out of the covers and onto his knee. 'Sorry, Em', can't be done. Here, you sit on my knee and I'll sing you a song.' He pulled her close, inhaling her still faintly baby aroma, 'No, sit still, what shall it be.' He began on a lullaby and rocked gently, watching as her eyelids drooped. He sighed when small snuffles indicated the fact that she had dozed off.

He sat nursing her for several minutes, before sliding her under the covers. This last infection had been a close call; thank God for antibiotics and Maria acting swiftly with the oxygen. He supposed he'd better up-date his former wife, not that she would care, but he wasn't going to give her the chance of saying he hadn't kept her informed.

He crept out of the room and nodded at Maria sitting quietly in the adjacent bedroom doing some fine knitting. 'I'll be downstairs, Maria. She's asleep, keep an eye on her, I've just got a phone call to make.'

'Si, Dottore,'

Josh went down the stairs slowly, working out what he would say to Lesley.

He sat at his desk and mentally prepared himself before picking up the phone and punching in the numbers on the landline.

'Lesley, its Josh.'

'Yes, what do you want?'

He sighed under his breath. 'I just wanted to let you know that Emma isn't well. But I've started her on antibiotics and she is improving.'

'She's your daughter, Josh; I don't care what you do to her.'

'No, she's your daughter, Lesley.'

'I would have put her in an institution as soon as she was born. Do what you want to her. I don't know why you bother with her, but you decided to keep her.'

Josh grabbed his slipping temper. 'Because I love her, Lesley.'

'Pity.' Lesley, at the other end of the phone, looked at herself in the mirror and wet a finger, smoothing down her eyebrow over light blue eyes. 'She's a freak, Josh, let her die. Now if you've got nothing more to say, I'm busy.' She laid the receiver back in the cradle quite gently.

Josh, a man not given to expressing his temper, nevertheless picked up a pencil and snapped it in half with his eyes shut, and a wish that it might have been his ex-wife's neck.

'*Hwrgi.*' He muttered the word and opened his eyes to see Joan standing in the open doorway.

'That, Josiah Blevins, is a word you didn't learn in this, or your father's house.'

Josh shook his head and sighed deeply. 'Sorry, Joan.'

'I suppose you were speaking to Lesley?'

'Yes, she makes me so...' He waved an expressive hand as words failed him.

Joan nodded. 'You're forgiven this once. How is Emma now?'

'We've caught it in time, I think, I hope, but short of a transplant, there isn't much I can do but keep the infections at bay and keep her happy.'

Joan nodded, 'Will you stop sending her to playgroup?'

'I've thought about it, Joan, but I can't wrap her in cotton wool. She would be miserable on her own. Better a short life and a merry one.' He spoke bitterly and Joan, after a glance at the expression on his face, nodded and left him, shutting the door after herself.

She and Maria, the nanny they had employed as soon as he brought Emma home, would cope for an hour or two. Joan didn't know all the ins and outs of why the marriage had failed within six months of the wedding. She did know that she thought Lesley a nasty piece of work.

Josh, left in the isolation of his study, stared at the broken pencil and ground his teeth for a minute or two. Women, he couldn't understand them. He'd made a hash of his marriage; Lesley had seemed to be as much in love with him as he thought he was with her. She said the baby she'd conceived was his, so he'd rushed her to the altar.

When little Emma was born with Down's syndrome and cystic fibrosis she'd totally rejected the child. He had tried; he thought she would learn to love her baby eventually. He had his wife checked for post natal depression. He offered inducements. They would go away until she was over the birth and then they could be a family. But no, Lesley didn't want anything to do with her new baby.

Emma had been very ill, requiring blood transfusions within the first week. And her blood work proved she wasn't his daughter at all if the brown-eyed baby of blue-eyed parents hadn't already given him a clue. Lesley wouldn't tell him the name of the father and she wasn't going to keep that freak, she said. That had ended the marriage. But Josh had fallen in love with the small crumpled face and the sheer grit that kept the baby fighting to stay alive.

He'd brought her home and installed Maria to care for her. He'd rejoiced when she'd hit the milestones every baby arrived at. The fact that she was a good eighteen months behind others was ignored. He loved her unconditionally, and found that love returned.

Now he smiled and spoke to the picture on his desk. 'OK, kiddo, dad will do his best.' He picked up the phone, speaking to the hospital switchboard. 'Put me through to the Mother and Baby Ward, please.'

He waited through a series of clicks, and then heard the familiar voice of Gill. He smiled to himself, 'Gill, Josh here, when is that nice nurse, Alexis, back?'

'Sorry, Josh, she took the weekend off, and I don't think she's coming back to our ward. She's agency, I told April to tell you.'

Josh nodded at the receiver, 'Yes, she passed the message on yesterday.' He frowned, of course Alexis had told him she was going away too, but he thought she'd go back to that ward after her weekend. While he was thinking, Gill waited patiently at the other end of the line.

'Josh, can I help?'

'No, it's not that important.'

'Well, while I've got you on the phone, I don't like the look of your Mrs. Cresswell. She's hardly stirred and she isn't eating.'

'Grief?'

'I thought so too, and didn't want to make too much fuss, but I'm just a tad worried about her.'

'Vitals?'

'Mild pyrexia and tachycardia. But lack of food and fluid could do that.'

'Anything else?'

Gill shook her head at the phone, and then said. 'No, it's just...'

Josh looked blankly at the other wall for a minute. 'OK, I'll pop along and take a quick look if you want me too.'

He went out of the study and took the stairs two at a time, coming into his daughter's room and looking at her in the small bed. Dolly was clasped in her arms, the mask was quietly hissing, though now the oxygen level was only at three litres. He spoke softly to Maria while he looked at his daughter. 'I've got to go to the hospital. Give the next dose of antibiotic at six, if I'm not back. I'll give the Panadol when I get in, she should hold for now. Let her sleep as long as she wants and don't fuss too much about food if she refuses it.'

'Si, Dottore.' Maria smiled at him. 'I will keep her happy for you.'

Josh nodded his head and left for the hospital. It looked like it could be a long night.

Chapter 5.

JOSH HAD BEEN RIGHT; it had proved to be a very long night indeed. Jane Creswell lay in the bed looking at the ceiling; she'd answered his questions politely enough but it was as if she was shutting out the world. He read her chart, examined her chest and looked at her husband for further enlightenment. Jock shook his head.

'I'll pop in tomorrow, see how you are.' No reaction. Not even a 'thank you', and that wasn't Jane Creswell. He jerked his head towards the door and Jock followed him out. 'Any idea, what's wrong, Mr. Creswell, aside from the obvious?'

Jock shook his head. 'She says she's not hungry. She snapped at me when I told her she must eat, it makes you feel inadequate, not fit for anything but a sperm donor.' He looked bitterly at Josh. 'I know she doesn't mean it, but it was my babe too, and...' He pushed a hand under overlong and uncombed hair, his eyes filling with tears. 'I seem to have lost them both.'

Josh nodded. 'Shall I arrange a grief counsellor for you both?'

Josh shook his head. 'We're not ready to talk to each other yet, how can we talk to a stranger?'

'Sometimes it's easier.' His lips twisted a bit

wryly. 'Let me know, if you do want someone. Both the staff here, and I, will monitor Jane closely.'

'Yes, alright.' Jock turned his hand on the door and then looked at Josh. 'I wish I'd had a vasectomy, I knew she shouldn't risk having babes but she wanted one, just one, so I gave in. But I'm going to book myself in, that way it won't happen again. I can't lose her too.'

Josh nodded and watched as Jock re-entered the single room. He was striding down the corridor when his mobile phoned. He flicked it open, 'Yes, Joan?' He listened to her for a moment increasing his speed until he swept out the main doors and headed for his car. 'I'm on my way, increase the oxygen again.'

Emma was lying over Josh's knees, at three the next morning. He was seated in the low rocking chair and he was patting her back in the rhythmic pattern taught him by the physiotherapist. She started to cough and choke, and eventually, weakly dribble mucus from her mouth. He wiped it away and lifted her up setting the mask back on her face. 'Better, *Cariad*?'

She nodded, tears filling her eyes, and her smile totally absent.

'How would you like to go with daddy to hospital for a few days?'

'No, no 'ospital, no needles, no, daddy, please.' She began to cry in earnest, the tracks from nose and eyes leaving dirty marks on the usually sunny face. Then the coughing began again. Josh upended her on his knee and pulled the mask away, patting her back until the sobs subsided.

He sat her upright again. 'Alright, *Cariad*, no hospital, unless we really have to. Go to sleep, Daddy's, here.' He rocked her gently and was rewarded by snuffles and snores within minutes. But her hand clung to his as she lay in his arms. Eventually he managed to slide her under the covers and sit back, watching her face and the struggling chest.

His daughter hated hospital. It usually involved IV antibiotics. They'd been lucky so far this last year, she'd been relatively healthy. The consultant paediatrician was aware of her case, but there had been no need to do more than have her shots and monitor her.

That was the main reason he'd moved up the county from Kendal. He was aware that she was nearing the end and he wanted the best for his daughter. This latest infection had caught everyone on the hop, however. Aside from the regular medicine and checkups she had seemed so well he'd almost begun to think he'd misjudged his timing.

He was still sitting, dozing in the chair when Joan came in at seven. She spoke softly, 'Go and get a shower and something to eat, Josh, I'll watch her.'

'Fifteen minutes.'

'I'm not going anywhere; take time to clear your head. You're no good to her if you wear yourself out.' Joan sat in his vacated chair and folded her hands placidly in her lap.

Josh nodded, but he didn't say anything, and

within fifteen minutes he was back in the bedroom, a mug in his hands. 'You are a lifesaver, Joan.' He toasted her with the mug as he came over.

'You need more than black coffee, Josh.'

'Uh huh.'

'How is she?'

'Very ill, she needs admitting.'

'Are you going to?'

Josh shook his head, 'I may have to, I'm going to set up a drip and give her some intravenous AB's here, but she isn't going to like it. I need to nip to the clinic to get the equipment. And I need a nurse. While I trust you and Maria, this needs a bit more training.'

Joan nodded. 'I love her, but I don't think I can give her injections, Josh.'

'Not asking you to, Joan. That's why I'm going to get a nurse.'

Joan smiled. 'Maria and I will get her washed and changed while you go and eat.'

Josh began to shake his head.

'Josh, go and eat! She's asleep. It would be better if you did your errands while she's sleeping or otherwise occupied. And you look like a pirate have a shave for heavens sake.' She shook her grey head at him, 'What would you patients say if they could see the elegant Josh Blevins at the moment?'

'You're right.' He sighed, 'Why do you always have to be right.'

'Comes of mothering you, lad.'

Josh gave her a lopsided smile and leant over to kiss his daughter. Then he went downstairs and ate a slice of toast while he stood in the kitchen waiting for the mobile to pick up at the other end.

ALEXIS RETURNED TO HER ground floor flat at nearly four that Sunday afternoon. Everyone had been to church and Sunday School. The lunch afterwards, especially the treacle pudding and custard, had even made the children a bit sleepy. They had played in the back garden, Eva washing dolls clothes and having a tea party for her dolls, with the somewhat chaotic assistance of Peter and the willing, if docile, help of Carl. Alexis had even managed a bit of sunbathing stretched out on a lounger, with the Sunday papers.

It had been, Alexis, paused in her thoughts as she pushed open her flat door and felt the heat of a late spring day hit her, it had been lovely, relaxing and homely. But Mary Down was right, she was hiding. In her professional life she was confident, independent and determined to get and give, the care her patients needed.

Her private life was another matter. She'd not been an easy child to take on, consumed with grief, in a land where she was teased and mocked for her funny accent. Her younger self had felt betrayed by her parents for leaving her, and betrayed by a system that did its best, but hadn't found her a permanent home for nearly three years.

She'd been bullied at school as soon as they realised she was a foster child. She had nightmares about finding her mother's corpse, remembering the cold stiff hands that hadn't responded to her frantic pleas for answers.

She had resorted to self-harming as a way of coping, small sharp increments of pain that brought relief for a brief period of time. The injuries had healed, leaving scar tissue on her legs. Hidden from everyone, including Mary. But then as she got older she had cut herself more deeply and more often. Until one day when Alexis was fifteen, Mary Down had been forced to take her to hospital to have the cuts stitched.

Mary had reproached herself, talking about how she'd missed the signs. But it had been the nurses who had really upset Alexis. They had threatened to stitch the leg without pain relief, because, they said, she evidently wanted to feel pain.

That had been a wake-up call for Alexis. Both Mary and she realised then that she needed counselling to cope with the trauma in her life. That had helped, and finally being adopted by Mary, and her husband, Ralf, had given her the confidence to cease inflicting pain on herself. Mary was right, she had come a long way from that small terrified child, but the inner scars could still hurt if they were knocked by events.

She had moved away from that home to study and take her degree. Ralf and Mary had come to see her capped. They'd supported her through the post-grad year and they'd cheered her on when she had said she wanted to specialize. Then Ralf had died and she had so wanted to take the pain of loss away but knew that way wasn't open to her anymore.

Now she dropped her overnight bag in the small lobby and scooped up the mail from the day before. She shed her coat as she passed through the sitting room, leaving it draped over the sofa back, and kicked off her flat loafers as she trailed into the kitchen. Dropping the letters on the countertop she went to the sink and filled the kettle, before putting a fruit teabag into a small teapot and rummaging in the tin for a chocolate ginger. She took a satisfying bite and hitched up on the barstool at the counter, picking up a knife left on the top and slitting open the first letter. She drew it out as she was about to take a second bite of biscuit. The hand holding it stilled as she read through the missive.

Ring me as soon as you receive this, as a matter of urgency, on the mobile number you will find below. Josh.

She turned the single sheet over and looked at the blank sheet on the back. Then re-read it, her lips moving with the words, 'No please or thank you, no dear Miss whatever, just a command.' She shook her head, 'I'll get to you, but I need five to drink my tea and unpack. I can't think of a single emergency, unless,' She paused as she picked up her mug. 'Unless it's one of the babies. Nah, there are plenty of nurses to care for them.'

She had barely lowered herself to the squashy sofa when there was a loud thump on the door and a finger pressed unremittingly onto the doorbell.

'Alright, keep your hair on, I'm coming!' She padded through the doorway and swung the door open.

Josh stood in her entrance. She looked at him in astonishment. He looked dishevelled, his normal suit replaced by jeans and a t-shirt, his leather jacket swinging open, he hadn't managed that shave and his chin was dark with a nascent beard.

He brushed past her before coming to a stop in the sitting room, he pointed accusingly at the mug on the coffee table. 'It's an emergency, but no, you just sit there drinking tea. You women are all the same, if a child isn't normal, isn't pretty, you won't lift a finger. Well you can get your coat and come with me, now. I don't care, Emma needs you.'

Alexis, following him into the room, edged past him and stepped away from the anger emanating from his body like a heat wave.

'I have no...'

She got no further; he picked up her coat and gestured to the door. 'I don't care if you have no intention of obeying me; you are coming, right now.'

Alexis sat down on a chair. She put her knees together and folded her hands in her lap. They were, if the truth was told, trembling, but it gave them both the illusion that she was confident she could stand up to him. She shook her head at him as he opened his mouth, and then lifted a finger. 'I was about to say I have no idea what you are talking about? I don't know who Emma is? I don't know why she, or you, need me, and,' she lifted her hand as he would have spoken over her. 'I will be damned, if I'll be accused of neglecting children because they aren't pretty! You know nothing about me.'

Josh shook his head. 'I haven't got time for this.'

'Until you explain a bit, I'm not going anywhere. Especially with some madman who has just invaded my home.'

Alexis folded her lips, raised an eyebrow and waited, watching him. He pushed a hand through his hair. 'OK, I'm sorry.' Alexis sniffed, she didn't think much of his apology.

He looked around as if for inspiration.

'Emma?' Alexis prompted.

'Emma is my daughter, she is very ill, Maria hasn't got the training to care for her when she is this ill. I need a nurse.' He pointed at Alexis. 'You.'

Alexis stood up. 'Right, I'll just get my shoes.'

'Shoes.' He looked at her blankly.

'Mr. Blevins, I have been back from my weekend less than ten minutes. I have removed my shoes and coat and brewed tea,' she glanced regretfully at the cooling mug, 'but I am prepared to come with you, but you should know...'

Josh was already heading out the door and she spoke to his retreating back. 'Oh well.' She sighed slightly, went into the kitchen, pushing her feet back into the despised shoes, and grabbed her shoulder bag in passing.

Josh was in the Jeep, the engine running, and her jacket slung onto the seat. She climbed in, and he waited impatiently for her to fasten up. He shot away from the curb as soon as he heard the click of the belt going home.

'You should know I'm not a Paediatric nurse.'

'But...' He glared at her, then swung his eyes back onto the ribbon of road in front of him. He addressed the windshield. 'Why were you working on the Mother And Baby Unit?' His voice might be calm, but his hands had the wheel in a death grip.

'Because they were short handed and that's where the agency sent me.'

'*Pentwp!*'

'I beg your pardon?'

Josh shook his head. Now he'd got her in the vehicle she could see he was calming a bit. 'What's you discipline?'

Alexis's lips twitched. 'Cardiac.'

'Yeah, I messed up there didn't I? Or maybe I didn't.' But he didn't seem to require an answer and both fell silent as they negotiated the late afternoon traffic out of the centre of the city. Alexis opened her mouth once as they swept past the entrance to the hospital. Then she closed her mouth again. She had expected to be taken there, despite his comments, but Josh pulled up in a cul-de-sac outside a Victorian redbrick house on the outskirts of Carlisle five minutes later. He switched off and came around the car, opening the door and waiting impatiently for her to climb down.

She followed him up a small garden path to an

impressive front door which stood ajar. He didn't stop on the threshold, but carried on straight up a flight of stairs in the entranceway. Alexis shrugged and, still carrying her shoulder bag, followed him.

Josh pushed open a door and they entered a little girl's dream bedroom. She noted in passing the Princess bed with canopy, a shelf of books, more dolls and soft toys than Alexis could count, and then focused on the small child apparently asleep in the bed. A pretty dark haired woman of about forty was sitting next to it, knitting.

The little face of the child in the bed lit up and a smile crossed her face, despite the hissing mask as she opened her eyes at the sound of the opening door. 'Daddy.' The little arms went up.

Josh went over, lifting her from the covers and into his arms. 'Thanks, Maria.' The woman smiled at him and gathered her knitting; she left the room on silent feet as Josh spoke to his daughter. 'I promised I would fetch Lexy for you; you have to keep your side of the bargain now, *Cariad*.' He rubbed her back. 'Dad has to put a little needle in your arm.' Emma frowned.

'OK, daddy.' Her lip trembled, but she held out her arm stiffly.

'Let's get you comfortable.' He went to put her back in the bed, but Alexis stepped forward.

'Hello, Emma. Do you want to sit on my knee? You can hide your face in my jumper if you want. It smells of my favourite scent - here have a sniff, while Daddy does the nasty business.' She took the little girl from Josh and sat down on a hard chair near the bed.

'Did you get any patches, Josh?'

He nodded. 'I put one on before I came for you.'

Alexis raised an eyebrow. 'And how did you know when I would be back?'

'I didn't. I've been nipping over every couple of hours since twelve this morning. You have no idea how relieved I was to get an answer to my knock.'

'Knock!' Alexis grinned at Emma, who was watching her father's preparations. 'He didn't knock, Emma, he was like the big bad wolf that blew the house down. He huffed and puffed and then he thumped the door.' She turned the little girl's face towards her, expertly imprisoning one arm and holding the other firm. 'Do you know the story of the three little pigs?'

Emma nodded; she tried to see what her father was doing but Alexis kept a firm hand on her. 'No, sweetheart, look at me. Dad will be as quick as he can.' She began to tell the fairy story.

As Emma felt the needle pricking her skin she began trying to wriggle and sob, but Alexis, expert at holding sickly foster brothers and sisters as she grew older, kept her still. She watched Josh securing the cannula in the arm and flushing it through. 'There, poppet, nearly finished.

'I'm just going to give you your medicine; you can watch that, Em.'

Alexis eased Emma around, smoothing the tears of the white cheeks with a thumb. Careful of the newly cannulated arm, she watched as Josh prepared a dose and had her check it with him, before he slowly injected it. 'All done. Good girl.' He looked at Alexis. 'If you could, er, sort things out, I'll be back in a minute.'

Alexis nodded, offering Emma a conspiratorial smile. 'I've got some sweeties in my bag. Would you like one to suck?' She glanced at Josh and got a faint nod. He left the room and she set the child down in the muddle of the bed for a minute. 'First the sweet. OK, Emma.'

Emma smiled, pulling at the mask. 'Wait a mo', poppet.' She found the promised sweet and handed it to Emma to unwrap while she looked around at the equipment Josh had left on the side table. 'Oh goody. Now, Emma, we have to make sure you don't undo daddy's work. You don't want another needle do you? So let me strap that arm to a splint.

Emma, sucking at the sweet, nodded. 'It won't hurt?'

'No, poppet. It stops it hurting, I promise.' She bound the arm up and then looked at the little face in front of her. 'Shall I make the bed and then sing to you?' Emma nodded again; she leaned back in the rocking chair while Alexis made the bed tidy and then gathered the child onto her lap and began to croon to her. Within minutes, Emma was asleep, the wheeze of her chest audible above the oxygen.

She eased the child into the bed, propping her up against the pillows, and looked at the rag doll from Friday night. She tucked that under the covers too and then set the room to rights. It was more than 'a minute' since Josh had disappeared out of the bedroom. She was longing for a drink of tea, but she didn't know where to go, and wouldn't have left the child if she did.

JOSH, AS IT HAPPENED, had received a phone call as he was going down the stairs. He fished his mobile out of his pocket and spoke into the machine. 'Yes, Blevins. Gill, what's the problem? Right, I'm on my way.'

He shot out of the house at a run. Joan, coming into the hall, saw his departing back and sighed. She turned around as Maria spoke to her. 'He bring, he brought, Lexy.'

'Did he, that's good, Maria. Is she with Emma?'

'Si, Joan.'

Josh had forgotten neither his daughter nor his new nurse, but Jane Creswell had risen from her bed and fainted. He didn't know what was going on, but he was going to get to the bottom of it now. He pulled up outside the hospital and, jacket flapping in the evening breeze, hurried along the corridor.

Surprising himself by how relieved he was feeling. He analysed the emotion while the lift took him up to the Mother and Baby Unit. He realized that for the first time he felt he could share the emotional care of his daughter with someone, and he hadn't known he needed to. He shook his head at the thought and then pushed all thoughts of his child to the back of his mind as he entered the single room.

'Hello, what's the trouble then?' He spoke to Jane Creswell, but also to the nurse sitting at the side of the bed.

Jane spoke from her prone position. 'I'm sorry, Doctor Blevins, they shouldn't have brought you in on a Sunday, and your day off.' She eyed his informal clothes. 'I only fainted.'

He nodded, sitting on the side of the bed. 'Why did you get up?'

'I thought I wanted the toilet, my tummy feels funny.'

Josh nodded. 'Have you opened your bowels since you gave birth?'

'Yes, and I'm peeing, the nurses keep asking about it.'

Josh only smiled. 'You aren't eating?

'No, I'm just not hungry, but I have been drinking.'

Josh nodded. God help them if she contracted the norovirus. 'Can I listen to your heart?'

Jane Creswell nodded sliding further down in the bed. Josh stepped back while the nurse helped her to lift her nightie, and then pulled the sheet up over her tummy.

Josh listened; the heart was steady, the new valve he'd transplanted the year before working well, the pulse regular. He listened to her lungs but they were quiet. 'OK. Let's have a feel of this tummy of yours.'

He tapped and palpated, starting at the left

upper quadrant and working his way around the abdomen. Finally he felt the uterus. As he gently pressed he was astonished to feel what he could have sworn was a kick into his hand. He moved his hand and felt again that tiny movement.

'Hmm, Nurse, would you be good enough to see if Mrs. Creswell's midwife is on the ward, and bring a foetal heart monitor back with you.' The nurse gave him an astonished look, and then swiftly left the room. Mrs. Creswell looked equally astonished. 'Just checking something, nothing to worry about.' He kept a hand laid gently on her abdomen while he waited and offered a smile.

He straightened as the midwife came back with the nurse. 'Doctor Blevins.' She gave him a nod. 'What's the trouble?'

'Nothing.' He smiled. 'Tell me, was the placenta complete?'

'Yes, of course, I would have alerted the surgical team if it hadn't been.'

'How's the discharge?'

'Scanty now, but Jane wasn't that far gone.' She frowned at him.

'I find the uterus somewhat enlarged.' Josh nodded, 'What do you think?'

'Well, it is a trifle, but not that much.' The midwife palpated the stomach and then stopped, her mouth forming a slight 'o' of surprise.

Josh looked at her. 'Yes, that's what I thought.' He watched as she spread gel on Jane

Creswell' stomach and switched on the monitor. The silent room was filled with the rapid beat of a tiny heart, beating steadily at over a hundred and twenty beats a minute. 'Oh my, twins.'

Jane Creswell, a quiet observer of these medical activities looked from one face to the other. 'Is that...?'

Josh nodded, a genuine smile lighting up his face for the first time that day. 'You appear to be pregnant.' He paused, 'Still.' He turned to the midwife. 'Why didn't we pick it up on the ultra sound?'

Jane spoke from the bed. 'Because I had a bad cold and you said, when I rang you, that they could postpone it for a bit, I've not had one yet,' She suddenly started crying quietly, the tears running down her face and making further words muffled, 'and I wanted one of those pictures to show, to prove to myself, I'd been pregnant, because it all seems a bit, as if it's a bad dream.' She sniffed and the nurse handed her a tissue.

'Well, you shall have a grainy black and white or even a three-d one if it can be managed on a Sunday evening.' He turned to the midwife. 'Bedrest. And arrange the scan please, as soon as possible.' He swung back to Jane Creswell. 'Eat. Little and often. We are going to watch you like a hawk from now on.'

ALEXIS WAS BEING OFFERED food too. 'Here you go, love. That man deserves a kick up the pants, fancy leaving you up here and not letting you know where anything is.' Joan shook her head as she set a tray down on the table at the side of the room.

She looked at Emma who was sleeping, her hands clutching the rag doll. 'Is she any better?'

Alexis nodded. 'Her temp is down a little. I've given her some more Paracetamol.' She looked at Joan who had appeared ten minutes before with an offer of tea. 'I didn't like to leave her.'

'No, of course you wouldn't, and if he'd used half the brains God gave him he'd know that. *Twp*.' There was a great deal of affection behind the words. 'Sit over there, and I'll rest the tray on your lap.'

'What does that mean, twp?

Joan smiled. 'Fool. But he isn't, not really.'

Alexis moved over to an old leather chair which would have looked more at home in a man's study. The tray was set on her lap and Alexis looked down on dainty sandwiches and a moist piece of rich fruit cake. The mug of tea was handed to her and Joan stood back. 'Enjoy that, I've put your suitcase in the next room.'

'What suitcase?' Alexis looked up in surprise, the sandwich half-way to her mouth.

'The one Josh left in the hall, love.'

'Oh.' Alexis finished the interrupted journey and put the sandwich in her mouth. She had no idea what Joan was talking about, but now wasn't the time to ask, she was starving. She grinned at herself round the second sandwich, and she'd had seconds of treacle pud too. She smiled nicely as she reached for a third.

'I like to see a woman eat, some of these lassies just pick, pick, at their food. It's a criminal waste.' Joan nodded at her and trotted off, leaving Alexis to wonder if the 'lassies' were brought to the house by Josh and that was how Joan knew about their eating habits.

She shrugged, polishing off the last of the sandwiches and looking at the cake with appreciation. She was just setting the empty mug back on the tray when Josh came through the door of the bedroom.

She looked at him in the light of a sunset that was turning the room's fixtures to gold and red. 'Oh, good, Joan fed you.' He walked over to his daughter and picked up a wrist, carefully monitoring the pulse and breathing before turning back to Alexis who had stood up and come over to the bedside.

Alexis nodded 'Yes, thank you. She at least seems to have thought about my needs.'

'Don't start; she caught me in the hall, I've had my ear bent already. I had to go in to the hospital.' He frowned. 'She seems a little easier.' He turned, picking up the charts he'd started that morning. Alexis's neat hand showed that Emma's temperature was down a little, and that Alexis had administered the evening meds.

'Settling in?' Josh was feeling uncomfortable, such a strange sensation for him that his voice came out more harshly than he intended. He looked at Alexis watching him and decided that what he needed was a kiss. Which was ridiculous, he hardly knew her. Then he decided he never would if he didn't get the kiss his body was now demanding. He took a step closer to her and inhaled her perfume. 'I am grateful. I was worried you see.' He edged a bit closer still. Her hair was like spun gold in the sunlight he thought. He reached out a hand and touched the braid hanging at the front of her left shoulder.

Alexis's hazel eyes widened as he boxed her in. 'I'd like to thank you properly.' He put a hand around the back of her head and waited, breathing in the same air, his eyes not leaving hers.

Alexis returned the look. 'Where's your wife?' She could feel her stomach clenching and her knees trembling slightly. 'Where's Maria?'

Josh lowered his hand, laying it on her arm. 'Maria is probably in the kitchen, and I'm divorced.'

Alexis felt the trembling move up to her chest as he lifted his arm again, and eased her head closer. 'Thank you.' He settled his lips on hers and waited for the world to stop spinning. He savoured the taste of honey and the smell of violets. 'Mmm.'

Alexis was left in stunned silence as he stepped back. 'Welcome to my house, Lexy.' He turned and walked out of the room.

Alexis flopped like a stranded fish into the low rocking chair and pushed the hair back from her face. What on earth was she to make of that? But boy, could he kiss! It wasn't as if she'd never been kissed before. But why had she responded quite so enthusiastically. She drew in a deep breath and then another, touching her fingers to her lips. She wasn't sure if she wanted to keep the kiss in or make sure of her own body.

She frowned, and who said he could call her Lexy. The man was altogether too high-handed. She had ten minutes to work herself up before Maria came in.

'I come help you bathe Emma, *si*?'

Alexis smiled at her. 'Yes she needs waking, she's due some more medicine and she must have something to drink too.'

Maria smiled. 'She a good girl my Emma. No trouble, always happy. She loves her papa, she good for him.'

Alexis nodded. Between them they lifted the little girl and helped her use the toilet, before putting her into clean pyjamas and sheets. 'Here you are, poppet, some juice. Just a sip and then we'll do a bit of physio, alright?'

'Daddy does that.' Emma was still wheezing as she spoke, and Alexis frowned down on the curly head.

Maria exchanged a look with Alexis 'I fetch il Dottore.' She sidled out of the room. Alexis lifted the child onto her knee.

'Want a *cwtch*.' Emma wriggled closer.

Alexis frowned at her, 'A what, Cherub?'

'She wants a cuddle, a hug.' Josh came striding in. He seemed to have showered and shaved since she last saw him. He certainly looked less strained. He gathered Emma up and Alexis hastily moved out of the way. 'One *cwtch* coming up, *Cariad*.' He sat, enfolding his daughter in his arms, and kissed her upturned face. 'Have you been good?'

'Yes, daddy.'

'That's my girl. Now, a little physio and you shall have a story, how will that be?' Emma nodded and he set her over his knee, face down, and began rhythmically to work his way along her left lung. Emma was soon coughing and choking, the tears, coming to her eyes. 'Daddy.' She spluttered the word out.

'Just a little more, *Cariad*.' He held her still with one hand while he tried to work her chest with the other.

'Emma, look, Lexy is having physio too,' Alexis crouched down and laid the rag doll over her knee and began to gently pat the doll. 'Oops, she needs her mouth wiping.' She continued to hold the child's attention as Josh finally brought up the congestive phlegm.

'There you are, Em, all done.' He set her upright and picked up the glass of juice. 'Drink, get rid of the nasty taste.' Emma's two hands gripped the plastic and she sipped, eyeing Alexis who was holding the doll between hers.

'Lexy needs a drink too.'

'She does indeed.' Alexis pretended to give the doll a drink and then tucked her under the sheets. 'She's worn out. I bet she falls asleep before I've finished reading you a story.'

She watched as Josh placed the child in the

bed and covered her up, setting the oxygen mask over her face. He indicated the chair he'd been sitting in. 'Story time.'

He stepped back, offered a half smile and moved over to the window to watch the last of the sun's dying rays as Alexis began a story about the princess and a pea.

Emma was asleep before half the book had been read.

Chapter 6.

'Would you come down stairs? I need to give you the background medical history.' He offered a half smile as he turned from the window. 'I also need your contact details for the Agency, since, if you're agreeable, I would like to employ you to look after Emma, for a few days at least.'

Alexis nodded her head and walked over to the bookshelf, replacing the book and straightening the table that they were currently using as a medical trolley.

He looked across to the bed. 'She'll sleep for a good two hours now, she's exhausted. I'll ask Maria to sit with her while I talk to you.'

He stood by the door, holding it open for her. Alexis glanced at his face as she walked past; getting a nice whiff of aftershave, but Josh's eyes had a shuttered look to them. She went down the stairs and waited at the bottom for him to join her.

She was captivated by the fittings and fixtures, especially a painting by one of the Dutch interior painters. Josh had rushed her upstairs so precipitately that she hadn't taken in her surroundings on the upward journey. Josh arriving next to her, caused her to heart to jump, she told herself it was because he moved so quietly.

He frowned as she straightened her back and stepped slightly away from him. 'This way.' He held a palm out and indicated his study before ushering her through the door and then turning away to shout down the corridor. 'Joan, I'm ready.'

He came back into the room and smiled. 'Joan's going to fetch us a cuppa to sustain us while she finishes getting supper.' He went behind the desk and said, 'Sit down, please.'

Alexis moved to sit in front of the desk, reflecting to herself that she wasn't so likely to make a fool of herself with four feet of solid oak between them. Joan, coming in with two pottery mugs on a small tray, frowned, sensing the strained atmosphere but not knowing the reason. 'Josh?'

He shook his head. 'Put it on the desk, Joan, and then give us half an hour.'

Joan glanced at Alexis. 'OK, Josh.'

She turned away and left, closing the door quietly behind her.

Josh nudged a mug towards her. 'I owe you an apology, I shanghaied you. My only excuse is that I'm rather desperate. Emma was working herself up at the thought of going into hospital, and I had this light bulb moment and thought I might persuade you to come and care for her until this crisis is over.' He smiled and picked his own mug up.

'If that's persuasion, heaven help us if you turn aggressive.' Alexis sniffed and took a sip of the hot brew.

'Yes, well, I've said I'm sorry about that.' Josh shrugged. 'I brought your overnight bag...' He grinned, 'more in hope than expectation, I have to admit.'

'Yes, Joan did tell me. I shall need to go home at some time in the near future, that bag has only got nightwear and dirty washing in it.'

'Ah, er, Joan could do your washing.'

'Do you ride roughshod over every one, or is it just the women in your life?'

'I don't...' He gave a soft laugh. 'OK, I plead guilty, but it's usually everyone.'

'Hmm.' Alexis sipped more tea and waited.

Josh set his mug down. 'Generally I keep my private life very private.' He held up a hand as the indignation and anger on Alexis face turned it pink. 'I am not suggesting you will talk, Alexis. I'm stating my position.'

'OK.' Alexis swallowed wrath and tea. 'I understand the need to stop the gossips, but Emma is...'

'Emma is my daughter and I am proud of her.' He nodded at her over his mug then took a deep breath. 'Now, Emma, she was born with Epstein's Anomaly, luckily or otherwise, she also had d-Transposition of the Great Arteries. The Epstein's allowed a degree of leakage so that the heart-body-heart cycle was circumvented. We operated in the first seven days and while we have re-routed the arteries, the heart is still damaged. You've seen the effect of the Cystic Fibrosis, which has exacerbated the cardiac problems.' Josh paused and sipped tea, moistening his throat. 'Her prognosis is poor to bad. She has perhaps a year at the outside.'

Alexis swallowed, feeling the desire to cry. She gulped more tea in order to shift the lump in her throat. 'She's a beautiful child.'

'Yes.' Josh drank some of his tea. 'Yes, she is.' He shifted in the chair. 'This latest, bout, I've yet to get the cultures back but it looks like a pneumonia bug. I've got her on broad spectrum Amoxicillin, as you saw. We may need to change that to something narrower, depending on the results. Though it does seem to be having some positive results now.'

Alexis, nodded. 'The oxygen therapy, does she have that regularly?'

'No, I got a tank after the last bout and kept it for just such an emergency as this. There's the inhalers, she's very good about taking them, the orals not so good.' His lip twitched upwards. 'She's only just five, I don't expect compliance all the time. Now as to her current regime...' Josh sat back and began to talk the technical jargon both of them were accustomed to use.

Twenty minutes later Joan appeared at the door. 'Supper, the pair of you.'

'Thanks, Joan.' Josh stood up, apparently relaxed. Alexis felt anything but, she hadn't done a lot of specialling and special of children not at all. Still it didn't look as if she was going to be left in sole charge of Emma. He led the way into a big kitchen with an

Aga in the corner jostling for space with a halogen oven and a microwave.

'Maria's had her supper. I'll just get the soup out of the *popty-ping*.'

Alexis stared at Joan. 'Popty-ping?'

'Microwave. Proper word, *meicrodon*, but half the Welsh population call it a popty-ping these days.' Josh held a chair for her and then sat down himself.

'So you're Welsh?'

Josh nodded. 'Yes, from Gwynedd originally, so is Joan, but we only use the Welsh when we're alone. It's rude otherwise.

'So you were being rude on Friday.' Alexis began to relax in the warmth of the kitchen and grinned at him, leaning back as Joan set a steaming bowl of soup in front of her.

Josh gave a half chuckle. 'I can't remember what I said, but I doubt if I was talking to you. This is called *cawl,* it's a kind of thick broth.' He picked up his spoon. 'There's welsh rarebit to follow. That's...'

'I know, cheese on toast.'

'Ah, but when you've tasted the real thing, its ambrosia. Not just boring cheese on toast.' He grinned at her and spooned up his *cawl* with enthusiasm.

'So, how is the wee lamb?' Joan at the other end of the table was eating her own meal.

'Improving, Joan, she'll need nursing for a few days yet, and keeping in bed.'

'And I suppose you are going to be at the

hospital, leaving us to deal with that.'

'I can come home...'

Joan waved a hand at him, 'I'm teasing you, lad.' She turned to Alexis. 'You've found your room comfortable?'

Alexis, thinking that her bedroom was nearly the size of her flat, nodded. 'It's beautiful.'

'And can you do her washing, Joan.'

'Josh!'

'Well, you won't ask, will you?' Josh looked across the table at Alexis. 'I brought her here in such a rush she didn't have time to pack properly, Joan.'

Joan nodded, standing up. 'Of course, it's no bother.' She moved over to the Halogen where the Welsh rarebit was keeping warm.

As they finished the meal Josh said. 'I know it's been a long day but would you mind sitting with Emma until midnight? I'll take over then, but I didn't get any sleep last night and I'm operating again tomorrow.'

Alexis shook her head. 'No, that's fine.' She watched him leave the room. 'Can I help with the washing up?'

'No, that's alright. I've only got to load the machine. Off you go and watch Emma. I'll come up and get your washing before bedtime.' Alexis was metaphorically shooed out of the room.

She made her way up the stairs and into the quiet bedroom. Maria smiled at her. 'She sleeps, the little one. I come if you need help.'

Alexis was left alone with Emma. She sat in the rocking chair and thought about what she'd learnt. Josh had taken her at her word and explained the child's cardiac problems very fully. What must it be like to know your child was going to die and you could do nothing about it? Especially when those problems were in an area you worked in daily.

Emma was a lovely child. Even ill she had shown herself to be strong-minded. Was she the product of a loving relationship? Why had her parents got a divorce? Consultants worked long hours. She supposed it could make or break a marriage, and a child with Emma's problems would make it even more difficult to maintain that relationship. But surely the mother would want to keep her, and Josh was a busy and important doctor.

Alexis frowned down at her hands lying still in her lap. Maybe Emma's mother couldn't cope with the knowledge of a terminal illness. Alexis could understand that. It would be hard not to get attached to the child sleeping in the bed near her. She sat for most of the evening, only getting up to wander about the room when she felt herself getting sleepy. She looked at the myriad of books on the shelf, pulling them out and examining the titles. At ten, she gave the next dose of AB's and checked the vitals. Emma slept soundly through it. Alexis sat down and relaxed, half dozing as the hours advanced.

Josh, coming in, saw her lying back next to the bed and thought how tired she looked. He felt guilty as he noted the circles under her eyes. 'Come on sleepy head, let's have you to bed. I'll watch her now.'

Alexis awakening from a light doze, looked at him with indignation. 'I wasn't that sound.'

'No, but I have no idea what you did today, yesterday actually. I don't know how long you've been up. And if I'm to make the best use of you, you need your sleep.'

'Peter rolled on me in the night, and it took ages to get back to sleep.' Alexis spoke absently as she looked at Emma. She missed the expression on his face, which went from astonishment to anger. She was a bit surprised to hear his voice become harsh. 'Then you'd better get your beauty sleep now.'

She looked at him, trying to figure out what was wrong. 'I've done her meds; she hasn't woken up.'

'Good, off you go.' He went over to the door, holding it for her, then, as she approached, scowled. 'I'd better give you a kiss in case you miss Peter.' The kiss wasn't like the last one in this room; it was fierce and demanding, sudden, and abruptly over. 'Good night, Alexis.' He gave her a gentle shove and shut the door on her.

Alexis shook her head; she couldn't keep up with his moods, what had she done now? She was too tired to figure it out anyway. She went to her bedroom, had a quick wash and brushed out her hair and, quickly stripping, got into a nightgown and slid between the covers.

Josh meanwhile was kicking himself. He sat in

the chair she had so recently vacated, looking at his daughter. 'Way to go, Josh, why don't you beat her up as well. Talk about jealousy!' He scowled at his hands. 'I don't know, every time I get near her...I...' He subsided, preparing to wait the night out.

It was three in the morning when Emma awoke; she was choking and turning blue in front of his face. Josh grabbed her up and shouted. 'Alexis.'

Alexis appeared at his side in a long t-shirt and little else.

'I need to suction.'

Alexis got the equipment from the table and held Emma's head still while her father worked at removing the blockage in her throat. The sucking sounds ceased and Emma took a breath, coughing and gasping; Alexis turned her over and hit her back with gentle thumps to shift the congested mucus.

'Intubation?'

'No, I think we've got it.' He took his daughter onto his knee, patting her back and wiping away the tears. He was, Alexis realized, not speaking English to the child. She pulled the rumpled bed together and went to get some cool fruit juice from the jug on the side.

'Here you go, poppet. Have a few sips.'

Josh took the glass from her and helped his daughter to drink then handed back the glass. Alexis noticed the beads of sweat on his forehead, and avoided looking at the tears on his cheeks. She looked away, 'Can I get you a drink, Josh?'

'*Panad* would be nice.' He offered a smile; it didn't reach his eyes as they watched his daughter falling asleep on his lap.

'OK. What's a *panad* and I'll get it for you.'

Josh shook his head gave a half choked chuckle. 'Cup of tea.'

Alexis left the room, and went down to the kitchen. She looked around and then, fearful of making too much noise, put the kettle on and found mugs and tea bags.

She crept back up the stairs with the mugs and went into the bedroom. Emma was sleeping, the oxygen a counterpoint to her wheeze as she lay in the bed. Josh was standing looking out on a moon-drenched garden. 'That was a bit too close for comfort.' Alexis took the mug over to him and looked out at the dreaming landscape.

'Yes.' She turned back and looked at the small girl in the big bed. 'She's breathing more evenly.'

Josh nodded and sipped from his mug. 'I'm sorry about the kiss.'

Alexis looked at him; he was grey under his night time stubble. 'Doesn't matter, Josh. You're worried silly and needing a bit of comfort yourself.'

'That's no excuse. I don't usually take my bad temper out on innocent bystanders.'

Alexis shook her head and he noticed for the first time that her blonde locks where unfettered and reached nearly to her waist. He also noticed the shortness of the t-shirt she wore.

He gripped the mug. 'Drink your tea and go to bed, Alexis, before I forget that my daughter is very ill and sleeping just over there.' He pointed with his chin.

Alexis took a quick glance at his face and what she read there had her setting the mug down and walking to the door. 'Good night, Josh. I'll relieve you at about six.'

JOSH WAS GONE WHEN she arrived in the bedroom, fully clothed, hair neatly braided, at ten-past-six that same morning. Maria was sitting by the side of the bed in her dressing gown, watching Emma. 'Good Morning, Miss Lexy, il Dottore he says, he will try to be back for lunch time and you are to go for walk then.' Maria smiled. 'We do the wash and then we play, si?'

'That sounds good, Maria.' Alexis nodded as she went over to the charts, checking the medication and vital signs. 'I see that Josh has taken her temperature. And reduced the oxygen to three litres again.'

'Si, she breathes better now.' Alexis came near the bed and smiled. 'Indeed she does, Maria. Do you want to go and get dressed, or even go back to bed for a little bit? I'll sit with her until you are ready to give me a hand.'

Maria nodded. 'I shower, now.' She patted Emma very gently on the hand. 'I not be long.'

Alexis was left alone with the sleeping child and her thoughts for company. She hadn't exactly slept well after she had returned to her room at half past three; the enigmatic man who had become her employer for the time being was giving her a headache. He blew hot and cold so often, she was going to have to see a shrink to cope. She sighed and sat down in the rocking chair.

She had been frowning at the opposite wall for several minutes when a little voice said, 'ello, Lexy, can I have a *cwtch*?'

'Of course you can, my poppet.' She swung Emma out of the bed and onto her knee, hugging her and smoothing back her hair. 'Are you feeling better?'

Emma considered the question. 'I want daddy?'

'Daddy has gone to work. At least I think he has.' Alexis rocked the warm body and dropped a kiss onto Emma's cheek. 'Will I do for now?'

'Now.' Emma suddenly beamed out a smile. 'I luve you, Lexy.' She began to pull the oxygen mask off.

'Well I love you too, poppet. But that doesn't mean you can do things you shouldn't.' Alexis placed the mask back on the little face. 'Shall we get a wash when Maria comes back in and then you can see if you want any breakfast?'

'OK, Lexy. Dolly too?'

'Yes, dolly too.' Alexis began to sing and rock as she waited for Maria to return.

JOSH WAS HAVING TROUBLES of his own. He didn't understand what was going on in his own mind. OK, so it had been a while since he'd dated, he paused there in his thoughts and frowned at the traffic streaming past his junction and into the town. Actually he hadn't dated since his divorce. In fact he hadn't had a woman in his bed since before Emma was born. He flicked his indicator and swung around a roundabout, heading into the hospital. Maybe that was it, a case of unfulfilled lust.

He parked in his usual slot and shivered slightly as he got out of the car; it was still cold for May.

He strode through the quiet hospital corridors still pondering his reactions to Alexis. Then as he reached his door decided he had better shelve the subject before he drove his self crazy. He shrugged; he would get the paperwork up to date, get a head start on the week. That would please his secretary and maybe settle his mind.

His lips twitched as he sat down behind his desk. Well, maybe not please her. He brought the young woman into his mind, she was bold and blonde and busty. She kept all comers at bay on his say so. She took no prisoners, when things hadn't been done properly. She was a treasure, and he had not the slightest desire to kiss her.

He gave a brief chuckle as he pulled a pile of files forward; just as well, her boyfriend was built like a brick outhouse and took no prisoners either. So why was he... he held his pen and stared blankly at the file for a minute... why was he lusting after a young woman who had offered him no encouragement at all?

Cardiac Arrest

He shook his head again 'No, that way lies madness and a very cross secretary.' His lips twisted wryly and he settled down to the paperwork, writing things in the margin of letters. Writing up his findings regarding Mrs. Creswell for the gynaecologists and obstetricians. He had spoken to them on the phone yesterday, but it was important for everyone to have it all down on paper. He would go and see her later he thought.

He pulled another file towards him and began to go through the notes of the patients he was to operate on later that morning. There were two pacemakers to be fitted, a CABG and an aortic aneurism that looked as if it might give soon and was better stitched before it tore. That one was going to be tricky, and he paused after he had read up the patient' notes.

His houseman had taken a thorough history, but hadn't tied up one or two symptoms with the presenting problem. Laying the notes down Josh frowned at the far wall where he kept current medical journals, before going over to his bookcase and pulling down a BMJ to check something he thought he'd read a few months ago. Hmm, it was definitely going to be tricky.

'Hi, Josh, you're in early.'

Josh's meditations were interrupted by the blonde dragon that ruled his office. She poked her head in through his door and smiled at him.

'Just checking something for later today, Sharon. Any chance of coffee?' She smiled, nodded, and disappeared.

Josh continued to scan the British Medical Journal, re-reading the article.

The coffee, when it arrived, was hot, strong and black. 'Thanks, Sharon.' He read to the end and set the mug down on the desk. 'I'll just be on the ward, thirty minutes, and then I'll be ready to scrub up. Let the theatre know, please.' Josh went through the outer office and tossed the words to Sharon as he disappeared out the door.

Sharon spoke to thin air. 'Sure thing, Josh.'

Josh didn't hear her; he was too busy pondering some signs and symptoms that he'd just managed to tie together. Monday mornings were always a bit fraught; the patients admitted over the weekend had a much higher risk of mortality than those coming in during the week. His housemen were good, very good, or they wouldn't stay on his team long, but they didn't always spot everything.

'Mr. John Cooper.' He stopped at the bed. The patient was a young man, thin of face, large of eye and wiry of body, he had been admitted with chest and back pain over the weekend. Ultra-sound had shown an AAA, an Abdominal Aortic Aneurysm; it was well advanced, nearly 5cm across. 'I'm Mr. Blevins, the cardiac consultant. I understand you're in Cumbria for a walking holiday.'

Mr. Cooper held out a hand. 'Hi doc, they've given me some pain relief and I still feel a bit woozy. The houseman said you might have to operate?'

Josh pulled up a chair. 'That was the original plan, but I need to ask you a few questions first.'

'Fire away.'

'Have you had any pain prior to this?'

'Nary a twinge, at least not in my chest.'

'So where do you get your twinges?'

'Well, my hips, knees and ankles ache something chronic, but what can you expect when I spend most of my life sitting at a desk. I'm just not used to the exercise.'

Josh nodded. 'Get cold fingers do you, lose feeling in them sometimes?'

'Yea, winter it's terrible. I've dropped no end of mobiles and as for using the computer...' John Cooper looked at him with a raised eyebrow.

'Tell me, Mr. Cooper, do you also have diarrhoea a lot?'

John Cooper looked uncomfortable. 'Hell, Doc.' He squirmed a bit in the hospital bed.

'Just answer the question, please. It's important.'

John Cooper nodded. 'Yeah, all the time, but then so did my mum. The doc says I've got IBS. I watch my diet, do all the right things, but it doesn't seem to have made much difference. Sometimes, I daren't go too far from a loo, it's that bad.'

'Hmm.' Josh sat back a bit. 'I think there might be a little more going on than a triple A. Mr. Cooper. I want to keep you in bed for a few days while I run some tests. I think you might have something called Ehlers-Danlos Syndrome; it's a connective tissue disorder which can range from difficult to live with, to downright life threatening. If you have, it will affect the way I treat your triple A. And the way I treat it now will effect how it will be treated in the future.'

'My uncle had a Triple A. He nearly died, but they just opened him up and stitched it up. Can't you do that for me?'

Josh slowly shook his head. 'If you have the syndrome the risk of open surgery is far greater than normal.'

'Oh.' John Cooper moved back in the bed and Josh could see a fine shiver going over him.

'Pain?'

'Panic.'

'OK, this is what we are going to do, I'm going to order blood tests and put a priority on them; if, in the mean time, the pain becomes worse, or I think there's a real danger of rupture, I will operate straight away. I know it's no good saying 'don't worry', but try not to. The nurses will be checking you on an hourly basis, any increase in pain, breathlessness, stomach ache, back ache or even leg ache, anything, you let them know straight away.' Josh stood up. He held out a hand. 'Let's hope I'm wrong shall we?' His lip lifted in a wry grin. 'I'd rather be safe and wrong.'

'Right you are, Doc. You're the boss.'

Josh nodded at him and left to go up to the theatres. Scrubbing up took time. He removed his signet ring and put it in the locker with his clothes, and then went into the clean room to start on his hands and arms.

His houseman, Harry Vincent was there. 'Hi Josh, everything is all set.'

Josh finished the minute routine and held his arms out for his gown, waiting patiently for the scrub nurse to tie him in and fit a mask. 'Yeah. I've decided to do a dual-chamber for Mrs. Otis. I think it will serve her better.'

'Did you see that article about the Nanostim pacemaker; the FDA still won't approve it. Say it's too risky.'

'Well it can be, Harry, the latest research shows a risk of perforations. The French are a bit anti as well.' The two men strolled into the theatre discussing various procedures, before they began the process of swabbing the subclavicular area of the elderly woman. Conversation lapsed as Josh began. He liked his operating theatre quiet while he concentrated on threading the leads through the veins and into the chambers. He spoke quietly, asking the nurse to adjust the light or angle the fluoroscope better, and then satisfied, attached both leads to the pacemaker under the skin.

'Right, stitch her up, Harry.'

He stood back, stretching his back as he watched his houseman finishing up the wound placing a small drain, and then a covering over the site. 'That should hold her; we'll set up the pacemaker with DDDR and cover all the options, stat dose of AB's to be on the safe side.'

Harry nodded.

'Wheel her away while we scrub, staff.' Josh walked out and threw his scrubs into the waiting bins and went into the clean room to start the whole process of cleaning and scrubbing his hands again.

He was tired and worried about Emma but none of those working with him would have guessed from his attitude. He was also concerned about Alexis. It wasn't a lack of trust, so much as the realisation that he trusted her so much it left him puzzled about his own emotions.

The morning progressed without any real drama as Harry remarked as they sipped a coffee waiting for the final patient to be brought up from the ward. You couldn't live in a permanent state of crisis, too hard on the nerves. He'd hoped to get some sort of reaction out of his boss; normally Josh would have teased him about either his lack of nerve or the fact that he lived on his nerves all the time.

'Josh?'

'Sorry, Harry, lot on my mind.'

'I thought the op's had gone well.'

'They have.' Josh set his mug down. 'Come on, last one before lunch.' He went out of the rest room and Harry followed, slightly mystified.

They were kept busy, searching for a decent vein for several minutes, but Josh lifted one eventually and laid it in the waiting dish and turned to Harry. 'Go on, make a start.'

'Who me?' Horror could be seen, and heard, even through the mask.

'Yeah, you, it's about time you did some work around here.' Josh stood back slightly and allowed Harry to take the main position at the side of the patient. 'Make a big enough hole; leave yourself enough room to manoeuvre.' He watched, saying very little as Harry did his first solo CABG. Then nodded as the young man closed the incision. 'Nicely done, Harry, we'll make a surgeon of you yet.'

Harry's shoulders visibly slumped as he stepped back to allow the nurses to apply the dressings.

Josh walked him out of the theatre. 'Great job. Let's go and have lunch while I talk to you about Ehlers-Danlos Syndrome.'

'Eh.' He looked at his boss. 'Aren't we going to do the triple A before lunch?'

'Probably not. Get changed and I'll fill you in on something I noticed. I probably wouldn't have spotted it if I hadn't read an article in the British Medical Journal the other month.' The two men washed, changed and walked off down the corridor to the staff canteen. The theatre staff knew where to find him, he had his pager, and teaching his houseman was as important as doing operations.

ALEXIS DEALT WITH HER small charge easily. She could see that Emma was improving; the antibiotics were definitely having an impact on the pneumonia. Emma was breathing much more easily and Alexis had swapped the mask for a nose cannula. 'There you go, Poppet, much more comfortable, isn't it?'

Emma nodded; she had slept for a great part of the morning, and Alexis wished she herself had something to do other than sit. In the finish she had asked Maria to show her her knitting and now Alexis was occupied making a small dress for the doll, Lexy, from borrowed wool and needles. It wasn't something she'd done a great deal of in the past few years, but she found, after a few false starts, her fingers remembered what to do.

This was unfortunate because she had hoped that working at the knitting might have occupied her mind as well. A mind that seemed to have been taken over by someone else. A someone who kept remembering the kiss and the feel of Josh's body pressed briefly against hers.

She got up every so often to check Emma's vital signs, marking the level of oxygenated blood and the temperature. The child was obviously exhausted by her overnight bout of choking. Alexis watched the pale face for a minute, laying down her work on her knee.

What must it be like to know your child had a terminal illness? Would you fight with everything in the arsenal, or let her go? If Emma was hers what would she do? Emma was never going to be independent, would always need care; unlike some Down's syndrome children she wasn't going to be able to leave home and have some semblance of an independent life.

Josh would know all the problems inherent in a transplant, the drug regime, the restrictions on life. Would Emma understand them? Unlikely. Alexis sighed; she didn't know what she would do. She could only guess at the heartache that Josh was going through.

She picked up the knitting and began to shape the skirt, muttering to herself occasionally as she had to take stitches back. It was a surprise when Maria came in and told her it was lunchtime. 'Joan, she says, lunch in the kitchen, Miss Lexy. I sit with Emma.'

Alexis nodded and stood up. 'I won't be long.'

'No, is OK, I have eaten. You go for walk like Dottore, he says. He not back yet.'

'Oh, thank you, Maria.'

Alexis, after a quick look at the sleeping Emma, went downstairs and enjoyed a light lunch and the company of Joan. After sighing and sitting back with a mug of tea she looked across the kitchen at Joan busy stacking things in the dishwasher. 'That was lovely, Joan. I'm not used to having such lovely meals prepared for me; it's usually the hospital canteen and a half hour to swallow it down.'

Joan stood up and nodded, 'Josh said you needed feeding up.'

'I don't really.' Alexis grinned. 'But it's nice all the same.'

'I'm pleased you enjoyed it, Alexis. Now we've to watch Emma while you go for a walk. Or Josh said you can borrow the mini that Maria and I use and fetch some more clothes if you want.'

'Oh. But...'

'I've Josh on the end of the phone, we know what to do.' She shrugged. 'If we have to do anything, but I'd rather not. I can't hurt the little mite, even for her own good, and nor can Maria. Pair of softies we are.' She looked at Alexis. 'I love her to bits; it's going to be hard when...'

'Yes, it is.' Alexis nodded, her face losing its grin. 'We'll get her through this episode I'm sure, she's improving all the time now.'

Joan gave a sniff. 'I know, Josh said. He wouldn't have gone to the hospital today otherwise, but he's fretting for her and Lesley...' She folded her lips together. 'Well, anyway, it's not easy being a single parent at the best of times. I'm glad he's got you to talk to.'

Alexis felt she should say she was only the nurse, not involved, something, but Joan had turned away to lift a set of keys from a rack near the back door. 'Will I show you where the car is, Alexis?'

FOR THE NEXT THREE days, the three women worked around each other so that they all had a break from the sick room. Emma was a child on the mend and wanting to do more than her strength would allow. The antibiotics were working well, and by day three Alexis had decreed that the Oxygen mask could be left off most of the time.

Cardiac Arrest

Emma allowed her to do the physio sessions and Alexis hardly saw Josh at all. He came home at lunch times while she was out for her walk, or doing an errand or two for Joan. She knew he was in the house in the evenings, but he seemed to spend most of his time in his study when he was there.

Emma chattered away in whichever language came to her first and Alexis had accumulated a small store of Welsh words with the help of Joan. She used them sometimes to cause Emma to giggle, and giggle she did.

'*Rho sws i mi*,' Alexis said the words slowly 'A kiss?'

Emma wriggled on her lap, dragging the towel from her bath time down and putting damp arms around Alexis's neck. She planted a wet kiss on Alexis's cheek. 'Me, me, now.'

Josh, standing at the door, nodded to himself. This was one woman who saw a child, not a freak. 'Can I have a *sws* too?'

'Daddy.' Emma beamed at him and held out her arms. '*Cwtch.*'

Josh came across the room and swung her, towel and all, up into his arms, squeezing gently. 'You're looking much better. I think tomorrow you might come downstairs and go into the garden. Mr. Sun has been waiting for you to come out to play.' He buried his face in her neck and blew a raspberry to cause her to giggle some more. Then he looked over her shoulder at Alexis. 'You'll be able to go home soon, Alexis.'

She looked at him with her head on one side; there was something different about him today. 'Everything alright, Josh?'

He nodded. 'Come on, Em, let's get your pyjamas on and have you into bed. Then I'll read you a story.'

The two adults working in tandem got Emma settled in her bed, and Josh began to read. He had both females giggling; the story was about a man searching for his cow, coming across various animals. Josh made suitable noises to match. He wasn't terribly good and that just added to the hilarity. But Emma's eyes soon drooped and she was asleep in the way of small children, suddenly and peacefully.

Josh leaned back against the bed head where he'd been resting as he read. He looked at Alexis, the smile still lighting her face as she rested in the rocking chair. 'I had an interesting case on Monday.' He spoke quietly, 'A patient who might just have EDS. He's in for a triple AAA.' He watched Alexis as she nodded her understanding.

'That affects the op' doesn't it? I saw one once. All that flabby tissue, means they bleed a lot more easily.'

'Mmm.' Josh nodded.

'Are you going to do an endovascular?'

'Depends on the results.'

'It's genetic isn't it?' Alexis frowned, trying to remember the details of her case. 'I can't remember if it's hereditary or familial?'

'Both.'

'Tough. Man or woman?'

'Man.'

'Well, at least he won't have to decide whether to carry children.'

'Would you?'

Alexis, faced with producing an honest answer, hesitated; but only for a second. 'If I was already pregnant, I couldn't abort. But if I knew the chances of something like CF was high, I might think twice about getting pregnant.' She offered him a thoughtful face. 'I'm a coward, I don't like to see suffering, and something as terminal as this,' she nodded at Emma, 'it's so heartbreaking.'

'Yes.'

'But she deserves to be cared for and loved while she's with us.' Alexis gave a half smile. 'Is that what you wanted to know?'

Josh nodded. 'Thank you.'

They sat quietly for a few minutes, then Josh said, 'Go and have a rest and a cuppa.'

Alexis felt herself dismissed in the nicest possible way. She smiled, leaning over and dropping a kiss on the nearest smooth cheek. 'Night night, poppet.'

Alexis looked at Josh. Josh held his cheek out to the side. 'Night night, Alexis.' Alexis leaned in and dropped a chaste kiss on his face, aware of the faint bristles and the smell of spicy aftershave. She felt herself blushing as she stood up and went down to the kitchen.

Joan, busy with the evening meal, smiled at her as she came in. 'Tea in the pot, Alexis, dinner in an hour.'

Alexis got a mug of tea and sat down in a Windsor chair next to the Aga, easing her feet out of her clogs. 'Oh that's nice, Joan. It's not that I've been on my feet much really, but it is nice to not have shoes on for a minute.'

Joan glanced over her shoulder from her position at the stove and grinned. 'Oh, I so agree.'

'I'll give you a hand if you want.'

'No, I've got everything under control. Drat!' The two women looked at each other as the doorbell rang.

'I'll get it.' Alexis headed through the hallway and opened the big front door, looking at the stunning woman on the doorstep. 'Can I help?'

Chapter 7.

'I WANT TO SPEAK to my husband. Perhaps you'd fetch him for me.' Lesley swept in and headed for the study. 'I'll wait in here. Bring me some tea.'

Alexis was left standing, looking at the inappropriately fur-clad back as Lesley sauntered across the hall tiles and closed the door of the study in her watching face.

Alexis stood in stunned silence for a second or two before going up the stairs and into Emma's room. 'Josh, there's a woman in your study; she says she's your wife and she wants to talk to you.' She dropped her bombshell and turned on her heel, heading to her bedroom.

Josh, after a blank look at the now empty doorway, laid the storybook down. 'Daddy will be back, Emma, I've got to see someone in my study.' He leaned over and dropped a kiss on the sleeping face. 'Lexy will be in to sit with you.'

He walked out and along the corridor. Knocking, he opened the door to find Alexis sitting on her bed with a blank look on her face. 'Could you keep an eye on Emma? I won't be long.'

Alexis stood; it felt as though she was moving in a fog. She watched Josh leave the room and shook her head. So, he had a wife, a past. She'd known that for a while, he'd said he was divorced, it didn't feel like it though, not the way that woman had walked in, over her, if she was honest with herself. And why should it matter? She was just the nurse, someone he'd needed in an emergency.

Alexis went along the corridor and into Emma's room. The child was asleep, clutching her doll, and with a smile on her face. Alexis went over to the window and pushed it open, drawing in a lungful of the soft, warm, evening air. The woman had worn fur. Why had she worn furs on a lovely evening like this? It could only mean she'd worn them to impress, and Alexis had to admit she had been impressed.

'Don't be so shallow, Lexy.' She muttered the words to herself. 'Just because she can wear diamond earrings on a weeknight doesn't make her any better than you.' She made a face at her own reflection, wisps of hair coming down, no make-up, and clothes liberally splashed from Emma's bath. She glanced down her person, 'Oh great! And I haven't got any shoes on either. How to make an impression on a man. And just why do you want to make an impression, my girl? Think about that.' She pulled another face and leaned further out

She didn't mean to overhear, she'd just wanted to take a few breaths, calm herself down. But the study was directly below the bedroom and the windows were open in both rooms.

'I want Emma.' The woman spoke in a strong voice.

'What do you mean you want her? You never wanted her.'

'Well, I want her now. I intend to come and get her tomorrow. She is going to live with me.'

'No, she is not.' Josh's voice was unnaturally calm, unnaturally quiet. But Alexis could hear every word of the sentence clearly.

'I need my child, Josh. I need to hold my baby girl.'

Now Josh spoke more quietly, and Alexis missed his reply as he said, 'Since when? Only a few days ago you told me she was a freak and that I should let her die, Lesley.'

Lesley spoke loudly enough for half the neighbourhood to hear, she sounded distraught, 'It's that thought, the thought of her dying; I need some time with her, before then.'

Josh was silent, he looked at his former wife, she looked unhappy, pale. He didn't know what to believe, but he didn't believe she had a maternal bone in her body.

'Josh, I have to have her, you've had her all this time, can't you let me have her for the last few months.' Lesley voice carried a note of pleading.

'No. she isn't a thing, a possession to be handed over. You can come and stay here, live in the house, enjoy her company, but Emma would be confused and distressed to be uprooted and planted in strange surroundings.'

'No. I want her in my house. You might have

custody but, she isn't even yours, you have no rights, she's mine and I'm taking her. I'll be back tomorrow.'

'You can't do that.'

'Yes I can.' Lesley stood up. 'I'll see you tomorrow, have her ready.'

'No, she isn't fit to be moved yet, she's been seriously ill. I've a nurse living in the house.'

'Then the nurse can just move with Emma, I'm taking her, Josh, and that's the end of it.'

Lesley swept over to the door and opened it, she looked back at Josh. 'Don't try any tricks, Josh, you haven't got a leg to stand on, and if you care for the child then you won't 'distress and disrupt' her life by being awkward.'

Josh looked at the closing door and put his head in his hands. He wasn't going to part with his beloved daughter, but Lesley was right; the courts might have given him custody, established his right to care for Emma, but morally his wife had rights to her daughter too. They had given her visiting rights and the right to share the child on an ad hoc basis. No court in the circumstances would grant her guardianship, but in the meantime. What the hell was he going to do?

He got up slowly, feeling suddenly older than his thirty-five years. He walked up the stairs, to find Alexis sitting quietly beside the bed, her hands resting in her lap, and her face devoid of all expression.

He glanced at the open window. 'You heard.' It was a statement not a question.

'Yes, sorry. I didn't intend to listen in.'

'Any suggestions.'

Alexis looked at him. 'Short of picking Emma up and taking her somewhere where her mother can't find her? No. And, is that the right thing to do, if her mother genuinely wants to have her.'

Josh lowered himself into the old leather chair in the corner. 'God knows, but I'm not about to put it to the test, right or wrong. Emma knows no other home but mine.'

'How can you stop her? A mother's love for her child can cause them to do all sorts of illegal things, Josh. She wants her child, and hasn't Emma a right to know her mother?'

'I can get a court injunction, tonight, to prevent her being taken away from necessary medical care.' Josh spoke slowly, thinking through his moves. Not really listening to Alexis. He glanced at her. 'You don't need to be involved in this. In fact it isn't fair that you should be. It will make it difficult in your career.'

Alexis looked at him. 'Are you seriously suggesting that I should just walk off and leave Emma to...to...' Words failed her and she shook her head at him. 'Do you really think I care about my career that much? You don't understand me at all.'

Josh watched as she stood up and came over to him. 'My career is something I love, but it's not the be all and end all of my life. I will not run away from this situation.' She paused. 'Unless you want me to go.

Do you?'

'I don't know.' Josh stood also. 'God help me. I don't know what I want anymore. Except... This could get very nasty, Alexis. You have to know that.'

'Yes, I know.'

He smiled. 'I'm going to call in a few favours.' His lip curled. 'I operated on a judge a few months ago, private patient, he's very happy with the rest of his life.' He smiled again, somewhat cynically, and left the room.

Alexis sat down next to the bed again. 'Alright, Emma, let's see how things pan out. We'll keep you safe, darling.' She went down for her dinner an hour later when Maria came to relieve her, but there was no sign of Josh.

Joan shrugged. 'He told me about his visitor. He's gone out, he won't be long, and you've to eat without him.'

Alexis, mystified, nodded and sat down with Joan. In truth she had little appetite for the meal but starving herself wouldn't help.

Josh came in long after she'd gone to bed. He found Joan sitting next to Emma's bed. 'Alexis says she'll take the midnight to four shift.'

Josh nodded, lowering his voice. 'How's Em?'

'She seems much easier now.'

He nodded. 'Good.' he paused, 'Joan, there will be a private security guard on the doorstep at six tomorrow, he is to see that Emma is not removed from the house. I have an injunction signed by a judge.' He waved a piece of paper at her. 'I've arranged for my houseman to do most of the rounds and take the first clinic, but I can't just abandon my patients. Hence the security.'

'Alright, Josh. We'll keep her here.'

'I'm not unreasonable, Joan, if Lesley wants to visit, then Emma is to be available, but she doesn't leave the house for any reason. Not to buy ice cream, new clothes, or go to the swings, anything, understand.'

'Yes, of course, Josh.'

He smiled. 'You're a gem. Now go to bed. I'll watch until Alexis gets up.

Alexis might have gone to bed but sleep was not happening. Was this, she pondered what Mother Mary meant by experiencing life? It was scary, she thought she knew something about Josh, was growing to like him more than a little, his obvious love for his daughter intrigued, fascinated and attracted her more than she wanted. She would have liked someone to look at her like that, hold her like that. Accept her with all her problems, so unconditionally.

But what kind of man kept a woman from her child? He must have loved his wife once to conceive a child with her. He needed to understand that not all people could face up to their fears, that having a disabled child was more than some women could cope with. Maybe his wife thought she had failed him, perhaps that's why the marriage failed, and it had been the thought of losing that child that had actually spurred her on to coming and demanding time with

Emma.

Josh seemed to be a reasonable man, but who knew what went on in a marriage. Maybe he couldn't forgive her for leaving; maybe he blamed her for the disability. Alexis sighed. That didn't seem to fit with the other things she had seen though.

She rose at the first ring of the small alarm on her mobile, pulling on jog bottoms and top over her t-shirt nightie and brushing her hair back into a pony tail. Josh was dozing in the rocking chair when she went in.

She gently touched an arm. 'Josh.'

He opened his eyes to see her leaning over him. His first thought was that he would like to see her hair spread over his pillow: the second that she looked very kissable. 'Hello, Lexy.'

She gave a wry smile. 'Hello, yourself. I think you should go to bed.'

'That's a hell of an invitation.' He watched the blush spreading over her cheeks. 'I didn't think women did that anymore.' He grinned at her but the smile didn't reach his eyes; those watched her shrewdly. He nodded at Emma. 'Much improved, temp is normal. I've taken her off the O_2 but use your judgment, if she seems to be getting short of breath put her back on it. I've written up the notes. I need to get a jump on the day tomorrow, so I'm going in early. I shall see you about midday, or earlier if it can be managed.' He smiled grimly as he stood up. 'Emma doesn't leave the house. OK? My ex is only allowed supervised contact.'

Alexis nodded. 'OK, Josh, but...'

'No buts. Emma needs to stay here.' He offered her the chair. 'Night.' He touched her cheek lightly with his fingers and left the room.

JOSH, TRUE TO HIS word, was at his desk in the hospital by seven the next morning. He had finished the paperwork and was drinking coffee by eight thirty, and, much to his staff nurse's disgust was ready to do a ward round before she'd got half his patients washed or medicated.

'Josh, really!'

He gave a grim smile. 'Sorry, April, but I've got things to do; I needed to check on Andrew Hardy. He's four days post now.'

'And I want you to have a word with Mr. Threadgold.'

April led the way down the ward and into the four-bedder that Mr. Hardy and Mr. Threadgold shared. 'Good morning, gentlemen.' Josh went over to Andrew's bed. 'I'd like a look at the leg incision, Staff, as well as the chest wound.' He spoke to Hardy while the Staff Nurse took down the dressings.

'How do you feel now? Any pain?'

'My leg feels sore, but other than that I feel really good.' Andrew Hardy lay looking at him; 'I would like to get up?' He voiced the question, his head on one side.

Josh shook his head slightly; he was observing the discharge from the chest drains. 'That can come out I think, Staff. And that one too,' he nodded at the healing leg. 'I don't want you to put any weight on that leg yet. It was a deep incision and I want those stitches to knit well, another three days.' He turned to April. 'Physio coming in?'

'Yes, sir.'

'The physio therapist is coming in; giving you breathing and leg exercise. You must do them.' He frowned down at Andrew. 'No cheating or skipping, it's very important.'

'You're in charge.'

'Yes, I am.' He shook hands 'I'll be back to see you in a couple of days.'

He moved over to Mr. Threadgold. 'Good morning.'

Mr. Threadgold was elderly, an ex sergeant-major, and inclined to ignore advice unless it suited him. Josh had asked the staff to get him out of bed the day after the operation. He was to be accompanied to the bathroom and sit with his legs dependent on the side of the bed at meal times. Mr. Threadgold was lying tucked up in bed and the breakfast trolley was fast approaching.

Josh stood looking down on his prone figure. 'I believe I asked the nurses to help you up, Mr. Threadgold. Have they not done so?'

The elderly man sniffed, 'Bunch of young lassies, I'm not doing what they say.'

Josh frowned. 'May I ask why not?'

Threadgold shook his grey locks. 'My legs sore,

I'm tired, and when I get home the wife will have me running about as if there's nothing wrong. I'm going to have a rest while I can.'

'Not in this hospital you aren't.' Josh spoke quite pleasantly, but firmly. 'You are to get up and use the toilet, not a commode. You are to sit out for your meals. The nurses are not here to wait on you; they are here to help you get well.'

'But Hardy there had the same 'op as I did, he's still in bed.' Threadgold scowled.

'Mr. Hardy's treatment is between him and myself. The same operation does not mean the same problems.'

'Now, you will get up! Do I make myself clear?'

Threadgold looked at the consultant and whatever he read in that face caused him to nod.

Josh nodded back at him. 'The nurses are here to help you, not run after you. Good morning.'

He walked out of the room to a silence that was as fragile as glass.

Once out of sight he looked at April and grinned. 'Give me a ring if he causes anymore trouble, the old so-and-so.'

'Yes, Josh.' She grinned back. 'That told him. I would have had an open rebellion if you hadn't spoken to him soon.'

'Yeah. How's Mr. Cooper? Have we got the results back from the lab?'

April handed him the sheaf of flimsies. 'His

white cell count is shocking, Josh. Neutrophils and Eosinophils are far too high. He's anaemic, less than 6; he has blood in the urine and faeces.'

Josh nodded. 'And the genetic test?'

'Not back yet; can you operate with what you've got?'

Josh shook his head. 'Don't want to risk it; he might bleed out on the table, look at these histamine and heparin levels. I'll go and have a word. I think we need to start him on whole blood, get a prophylactic AB on board. I'd like a scan arranged for the lower bowel and kidneys. Today if possible.'

'I'll try, Josh, but it's Friday.'

He nodded. 'Yeah. Do what you can, April.'

He walked into the small ward where John Cooper was sitting up reading a hefty tome.

'Mr. Cooper, John, how are you today?'

'Bored, but to be honest, I keep falling asleep, so not that bored.' He gave a small smile. 'Are you going to operate?'

Josh shook his head. 'Maybe next week. I'm pretty sure you have got EDS. Your blood work certainly points that way. I'd like to get you fit for the operation, so unless you have any objections I've asked the staff to give you at least three litres of whole blood.' He waited, head on one side.

'No, that's OK. Blood's well screened these days.'

'I also want some more tests.' He offered a faint grin at the theatrical groan. 'Not needles and blood, just a scan. They did one over the abdomen for the suspected the triple A, didn't they?' He waited for the nod. 'I want one of your lower stomach and kidneys as well.'

John Cooper nodded.

'If you have got EDS I shall need to operate using something called endovascular repair. It carries less risk during, and immediately post, surgery but long term there are more complications. We are monitoring your aneurysm and it is slow growing, we can wait, but I don't want to wait too long.' He waited for the nod of understanding.

'Once we have dealt with the immediate problem I shall bring in a specialist to help you understand your condition.'

'What's the cure?'

Josh shook his head. 'No cure, we can manage the problems but not fix it. I'm sorry.'

'Not as sorry as I am.' He took a deep breath, 'What am I going to tell my girl? She's three months gone and we're planning on getting married.'

Josh sighed under his breath. What would he have done if he'd known about Emma's CF before she was born? Would he have urged termination? He just didn't know and he wasn't sure how to advise this young man and his future wife. 'I'll arrange a meeting with the consultant and both of you. Explain the genetic chances and the risks for the child. OK?'

'Yeah. At least you spotted the problem before I dropped dead, this way I can at least make arrangements for her.'

Josh nodded. 'That would be as well. Not to put too fine a point on it, would you like me to see about getting you a solicitor too?'

He watched the already pale face turn milky-white. John Cooper looked at him. 'Seriously?'

'Seriously. Aneurysms are unpredictable at best.'

Cooper's shoulders slumped and then lifted, and he took a deep breath. 'Right, do that for me, Doc, and can one of the nurses call my girl, tell her to come in. I think we've got things to discuss.'

Josh smiled. 'OK.' He offered a hand. 'I'll be back on Monday and see how you are then. He turned and walked away. He spoke to April at the desk, setting things up for John Cooper. Then, pulling out his mobile and speed-dialling he strode off towards the bank of lifts. 'Joan.' He spoke quietly as he walked along the corridor. 'Has my security arrived? Good. How about Lesley? No. *diolch byth.*'

He went into the lift and closed the door, shutting himself in. 'How is Emma?'

Joan on the other end of the line glanced across the room to where Emma was busy colouring in a picture of a princess, with the assistance of Alexis.

'She's doing OK, Josh, she keeps saying she wants the needle out now.'

Josh considered; it was true the course of IV antibiotics had finished and she was taking them in a syrup formula now, but the cannula lent colour to his tale of a very sick child. He was weighing the medical needs of the child against the emotional blackmail he could exert on his ex-wife. But the doctor in him won without a struggle. 'You'd better ask Alexis to remove it.'

'Right, when will you be back?'

The lift stopped and wheezed its doors open. 'As soon as I can.' Josh nodded at a couple of nurses who had just stepped in. 'Ring me, as soon as you have company.' He flicked the little machine shut and smiled at the women.

He got off at the next floor and walked along to his day clinic; Harry was examining a young woman in one of the cubicles. He stepped out and looked his boss over, a worried frown on his face. 'I didn't expect to see you, Josh. Thought you'd got some urgent business?'

'I just stopped by on my way out, everything going OK?'

'No problems, so far, it's mainly call-backs and routine stuff today.'

Josh nodded. 'You can do it with one hand tied, Harry. Trust your instincts, man.'

Harry nodded.

'I'm at the end of the phone. But you can manage without me, fine.' Josh offered a nod in return and strode out of the clinic and into his car. He wasn't looking forward to the upcoming meeting with his ex but the sooner he laid down the ground rules the better for everyone.

It was a peaceful scene that greeted him when he returned home. He'd passed the security guard sitting on a hard chair looking at the paintings in the hall, for all the world as if he was at an art gallery. His daughter had moved on from colouring and was playing with her dolls, pushing them about in a doll's pram in the sitting room. The French windows were open onto the lawn and the sun was pouring heat onto the patio.

'Hello, *Cariad*. I see Lexy has taken out the nasty needle. That's a nice plaster, what's it got on it?'

'S'pitcher, Daddy, Lexy said it's a duck.'

'Yep, looks like a duck to me.' He glanced across the room at Alexis sitting next to the window. She looked so... he nodded to himself, so right there. 'Alexis, no problems?'

Alexis shook her head, but he didn't get the smile he expected. 'Do we have to have that man in the hall, Josh?'

'Yes.' Josh spoke harshly.

'But is it fair, your wife just wants time with her daughter. Emma should have the opportunity to see her.'

'I'm not stopping her; she can have all the time she wants. But she isn't taking Emma.'

'Isn't that a bit selfish?' Alexis tried to speak gently, but she had seen the fallout effect of too many broken marriages. Her foster mother had had to cope with the children left bewildered and blaming themselves for the separation of their parents. It was easier on the children if the parents could be at least civilised, in front of them.

Josh shook his head. 'You have no idea what my wife is like.'

'No, I'm sorry; I don't mean to interfere but...'

'Then don't. If you don't like the situation then you'd better go. Em' doesn't need you to stand up for her, she has me. Thank you for you help.' Josh picked Emma up and walked out of the room. He nodded to the guard and went into the kitchen. He hadn't meant to snap, but he was worried and distracted. He would go back and speak to her in a minute.

Alexis looked blankly at the still swinging door to the sitting room. She had never been so efficiently dismissed in her life. She rose slowly and walked up to her bedroom. By the time she had reached it the tears were dripping off her cheeks. She packed, throwing items into the small suitcase any-old-how. The tears had dried by the time she walked back down the stairs. In fact she was so angry she could have hit someone, and she had never hit anyone in her life before.

She nodded at the security guard and walked out of the door. She stood on the street, looking around her. The case wasn't heavy but she had no transport. She set off for the nearest bus stop, sheer fury propelling her along the roadway.

Chapter 8.

SHE ARRIVED HOME STILL with a full head of steam, but having run out of new words to call Josh, 'Arrogant, pig-headed, overbearing, selfish, swine.' She muttered the litany of words as she wrestled with the key to her front door. 'Boor,' she said as she walked into the flat. 'How could he...grr!' She flung her case down and then lifted her head at the chuckle coming from the kitchen of her flat.

'Well love, I know I told you to get a life and allow yourself to feel, but don't you think you might be running before you can walk.' Mother Mary walked out of the kitchen, Peter balanced on her brown, trouser clad hip. 'I had to come into Carlisle for some new shoes for this young man, and thought I'd pop in since you haven't been answering your mobile.'

One eyebrow raised as her daughter looked at her in astonishment and then burst into fresh tears. 'Like that is it?'

Mary set Peter down on the floor and went over, putting her arms around Alexis, the soft and comforting wool of the green jumper she wore receiving a few more angry tears. 'Come on, love, what's he done?' She paused. 'Or not done for that matter?'

Alexis hiccupped and sobbed, and wiped her hands across her face. 'Who said it's a man?'

'You did, actually, when you came in the door, but this much angst? It's got to be a man.'

'Oh! I'm so angry with him.'

Mary wisely kept her thoughts to herself. She led the sobbing Alexis into the kitchen, gently pushed her onto a stool, and swung around to the kettle. She poured water into the teapot and then tore off a piece of kitchen roll, holding it and waiting for the storm to pass.

'Right. Use this and then tell me who's done what to whom and when.'

Alexis busy mopping and muttering, sniffed mightily, and Mary pulled off a second sheet of paper and handed that to her as well.

'Alright, better now?'

'Yes, Mother.' Alexis accepted the mug of tea pushed her way. Mary walked into the sitting room, returned with Peter, and set him on the floor with a biscuit.

'Talk to me, love.'

'He told me to go, just like that. I thought he liked me, but all he cares about is getting his own way. She's not a possession, like a fridge or some records they have to divide up, she's a human being. Just because she couldn't handle disability doesn't make her a bad mother.'

Mary held up a hand. 'I have no idea what you are talking about, Alexis. Start again and this time, try for a little coherence please.' The bracing tones had the desired effect.

Alexis gave a watery chuckle. The tone was so reminiscent of her childhood. 'Sorry, Mother Mary.' She took a deep breath and started to explain. 'So you see I was trying to help him and show him another point of view, but he just chucked me out.'

Mary sipped her cooling tea. 'I hear what you are saying, love, but there's a deal of speculation in there. You really don't know why the marriage failed. They might have hated each other, his work might have been too demanding to make things work, she might not have wanted the child. We don't know.'

'But she said she wanted to have Emma.'

'And you don't know her motives.'

'But... You're right, Mother Mary, I'm sorry and he was right, I was interfering, bringing my own baggage to the problem.'

'No harm in that if you can help. But he must be worried silly about his child, coping with her illness. The last thing he needs is your reproaches.'

Alexis sighed. 'I think I've made a fool of myself.'

'Won't be the first, or last, time for any of us.'

'No.' Alexis squared her shoulders. 'I'll go and apologise.'

'I should leave it for now; let him get the meeting with his wife over, sort out the visiting rights, let the situation calm down.' She paused to think. 'Come home for a few days if you want.'

JOSH MEANTIME HAD ALSO tried to calm down. He'd gone back to the sitting room after he'd located Maria and settled Emma with her, but it had all taken time. By the time he got there Alexis had packed and gone. 'Blast, all women.' The security guard gave him a wry grin as he came out of the sitting room. 'Where did she go, the blonde?'

'Out. Took her bag and headed off up the road.'

Josh scowled at the door. There was a loud thump and the door bell rang. 'Oh shit, more trouble.' He stepped towards it and opened it to reveal his ex-wife. 'Great, just what I need.'

Lesley pursed her lips. 'Still as polite as ever I see. I've come for Emma.'

Josh shook his head. 'Oh, no you haven't. You can visit, I can't stop you, but you'd better read this before you go any further.' He held out the court injunction.

Lesley brushed the paper aside. 'I'm coming in.'

'Have I said I would stop you?' He followed her along the corridor until she stopped at the sitting room and peered into its empty depths. 'Where is she?'

'Emma is with Maria in the garden. She's playing in the sandpit, and if I might advise you, those clothes don't go with sandpits.' He looked at the taupe three quarter length trousers and low cut cream blouse.

Lesley ignored him and went through the French windows to where Emma could be seen sitting in the sand pit under a sunshade. She was dressed in a pair of dungarees and a red jumper and Josh looking at her as he emerged through the windows, after his ex, thought she looked adorable.

Emma was methodically filling a bucket with sand and tipping it out again.

Her mother stood poised on the edge of the sand pit and spoke to her. 'Emma.'

The child looked up and grinned. 'Ello, who are you?'

'I'm your mummy.'

Emma smiled at her, but then saw Josh. 'Daddy, I's making sandcastles.'

'Josh, I want a seat.' Josh gave her a look of dislike but hooked a deck chair and pushed it near the sandpit.

Lesley sat down. 'Come here, Emma, I want to hold you.'

Emma ignored her. 'Where's Lexy, Daddy.'

Josh, thinking he wished he knew, said. 'She's gone out, darling, will you sit on mummy's knee.'

Emma ignored this too. 'I want to show Lexy I can make sandcastles.' Her lip pouted.

Lesley, bored with this interchange and tired of waiting, moved and bent to pick Emma up.

Emma was tired; she had been awake all

morning for the first time in a week. She objected to being picked up when she didn't want to be. When Lesley accidentally squeezed the site of the cannula, Emma turned into a wriggling, screaming ball. 'Wanna play, don't like you. Daddy!' Were the only words Lesley could make out.

Emma was sobbing in earnest by now, tears, dribble, and mucus from her nose were mixing equally on her cheeks and transferring themselves to the cream blouse.

'Oh, you dirty little animal.' Lesley pushed her away so that Emma slithered onto the stone of the patio.

Josh picked Emma up, soothing her and ignoring the mess on his suit. 'OK, *Cariad*.' He murmured to her in Welsh, soothing her and eventually handing her to Maria. 'Put her to bed for an hour. I've promised I'll come up and read to her soon.'

Lesley stood up as Maria went away with the still teary child. 'That was your fault. You could have prepared her for me. She didn't know who I was, she was frightened. That's typical of you, Josh.'

'I think we need to talk, Lesley.' Strangely Josh was now calm; his temper throttled back. A small part of him was incandescent with rage at his daughter being called an animal. Another part of him was seeing Lesley more clearly than the day before. 'Study. I'll get Joan to fetch us some coffee.'

'I don't want any.' But Lesley moved indoors and followed Josh to his study.

'Why do you really want our daughter?' Josh barely gave her time to sit down. 'Let's have the truth instead of the load of bollocks you fed me yesterday.' He sat behind the desk.

'I'm pregnant.'

Josh had expected several reasons but that hadn't been one of them. He opened his mouth and shut it again.

'My boyfriend has got pots of money. He knows I've had a child before because he insisted on coming to the obstetrician. I don't think he believed I had a child in here and I don't think he'll marry me if I'm not.' Lesley patted her stomach. 'But I had to give my gyne' history.'

She paused to gulp air, 'He wants Emma; he says he'll love her. He says it isn't natural not to have her living with us, with me, her mother. He won't marry me if he thinks I'm not a fit mother. But he will take this baby.' Lesley touched her stomach again, and then looked at Josh across the expanse of desk. 'I thought Emma might be more human now. I thought I could cope with her.'

'Emma is human and If you say one more thing about her I swear I will throw you out of this house, pregnant or not.' Josh gritted his teeth.

Lesley sniffed. 'I don't know what to do. I thought you'd be pleased to be rid of her.'

'No, I love my daughter very much; I frankly don't know how I'm going to cope when she dies.'

'She isn't going to die yet, is she?'

Cardiac Arrest

Josh looked at her; did she want Emma to die? That last, 'is she?' had sounded more hopeful that worried.

'Can't you get her a transplant? You've got lots of connections, you could move her up the list and then she would be better. More hu...' Lesley stopped speaking at the look on his face.

'Emma would still have Down's Syndrome, even if she had a transplant. That isn't going to change. She is not a candidate for transplant, we've talked about this. She couldn't cope with the medication or the regime a transplant patient has to go through. Her other organs are beginning to fail because of the strain her heart is putting on them.'

Lesley looked at his impassive face. 'I thought you said you loved her. How can you talk like that, as if her death didn't matter? She's mine too and I say we should try to get her a transplant.'

'No. And you won't find a doctor prepared to do it. She is too fragile and always has been. We will not discuss this again, Lesley. I have guardianship of Emma and I have made the decision.'

'I could take you to court. Get the custody overturned.'

Josh sighed, brushing his hands over his hair and looking at the woman opposite. 'It would be an academic exercise, Lesley; she has very little time left.' He looked away for a moment, as he looked back at her face he struggled to interpret the sly grin. 'What do you want me to do?'

'Tell my boyfriend I'm a good mother. That it's not my fault you got custody.'

'And what will you do if you have another Down's baby? There's a chance, you're over thirty, and I presume you've worked out who has the cystic fibrosis gene, you or Emma's biological father.'

Lesley shook her head, ignoring the comments and answering the question. 'I won't have it. I'm booked for amniocentesis next week. If it is another one like that, I shall get an abortion.'

'How does the boyfriend feel about that?'

'I haven't told him. It's my body, Josh.'

'You are a heartless woman. I will not give Emma to you and I will not lie to your rich boyfriend. Tell him what you like.'

Josh stood up, 'Get out.'

'But...'

'Get out, before I do something we shall both regret.'

'You've changed, Josh, you would do anything for me once.'

'I've learnt sense.' He stepped from behind the desk and Lesley took a look at his face and walked over to the door.

'I shall tell him you are a selfish pig who is depriving me of my daughter. We'll see what he says about that.' She went out, nodded to the security guard, closing the front door with a click behind her.

Josh sat down again. 'Oh God. What am I

going to do when you die, Em?' he whispered the words to the empty room. He leaned back in his chair and closed his eyes, holding in the tears of grief by brute force.

ALEXIS HAD REPACKED HER bags, Mary had taken control of her dirty washing, throwing it into her own car boot, and Alexis had climbed into the blue Ford Focus and followed her adopted mother back to Whitehaven.

She addressed the windscreen as she pulled up outside the familiar house. 'I'm a fool. I should have gone back and talked to him. Said I was sorry. Mother Mary would say I needed to look at my own motives.' But she went indoors anyway and spent two days playing with the children on the beach and relaxing. And thinking.

TUESDAY SHE WAS BACK in Carlisle being addressed by the young woman at the agency. 'Hello again, I see they've found the source of the norovirus; one of the cleaners is a carrier. She was so upset when the results came back positive.'

Alexis nodded. 'Poor soul. Have they found her other work?'

'The hospital tells me they've moved her to office duties instead of wards.'

Alexis gave another nod. 'Not much agency work needed at the infirmary then.'

'Oh no, Miss Bowen, I can always place people

like you, I can even get you a cardiac placement.'

Alexis shook her head. 'No, something else please.'

'But you said you wanted cardiac.'

'Well, now I don't. I'd like something in one of the nursing homes.'

'You're rather overqualified for those.'

'Are you telling me that elderly people don't deserve the very best of care?'

'No, no, of course not, but we could find you work in one of the more challenging placements where all your skills could be used to good effect.'

Alexis shook her head. 'The last job was quite challenging enough for me, thank you.' She smiled nicely. 'I'd like something not quite so demanding for a few weeks.'

'There's always places in the nursing homes, a lot find it boring, or just too physical. I can find you work with no trouble. It's night shift though?' She printed an address out, but as she handed it over she gave Alexis a worried look. 'Did Mr. Blevins find you? He came to us yesterday. Said you'd taken a couple of days off as is your right, but he'd like you to continue working for him.'

Alexis paused. 'Is it his daughter again?'

'He didn't say. I expect so.'

'I'll take this job, but I'll contact you if I need to change, will that be alright?'

She got a nod of agreement. 'He was very

complimentary about your work, Miss Bowen.

Alexis nodded back. 'Always good to know.' She left the agency and went into the city centre, pondering what she should do. She had, 'thought about her motives'. She found she was scared of staying around the child because she had become very attached to her in a very short time. But worse than that, she discovered her heart wasn't as whole as she'd thought and the man who'd made the inroads was Emma's father.

Alexis considered he'd got enough problems without a nurse falling for him in classic medical romance style. She had heard the gossip, while she was still up on the mother and baby unit.

He'd even told her himself, he didn't want her getting too involved or chasing him. He hadn't said it in the manner of a man proud of his conquests; it had been said in exasperation. She would walk away while she still could. She wasn't running or hiding she assured herself. Just playing safe.

She finished the cup of coffee she didn't want and went home, doing a little needful shopping on the way. She needed to catch a couple of hours sleep if she was to go on shift at nine that night.

She checked that she knew where she was going, before drawing the thick curtains and crawling under the feather duvet. It wasn't going to be easy getting to sleep when the daylight was still there at ten at night.

By eight she was on her way to one of the private nursing homes in the centre of the city. She took notes at the handover and went around the rooms introducing herself and wishing the patients 'good evening' as she helped them with their medication.

'It looks like it should be a quiet night.' She spoke to the two carers after they finished getting the last of the residents into their nightwear.

'Oh, it's not too bad, we've got one or two hang on the bell, they usually want the toilet; sometimes they just want a bit of company when they can't sleep. But most of them are OK.' The woman brushed untidy hair out of her eyes with a reddened hand. In build she would have made two of Alexis. 'We generally have a cuppa about now, and then the bells start for the first round of toileting. It goes quiet then until gone midnight, you'll see.'

Alexis smiled nicely. 'Fine, you keep me straight; you know them better than I do.'

The night moved along; those who had been acting as carers for many months knew the residents well. Alexis found her biggest problem was staying awake. She lent a hand, and sometimes some muscle, when it came to getting people up for the toilet. The carers where more than capable most of the time using their sturdy bodies to hoist and lift.

She stripped beds after 'accidents'. She made tea and sat with elderly women who had spent the bulk of their lives sleeping next to their husbands and now couldn't sleep, because the small divan was just too big and the room too quiet. By six in the morning, she was more tired herself than if she had done a full-on shift in A & E. A different kind of tiredness; emotional rather than physical she thought.

'I'm just going to get a coffee.' She smiled wryly at the senior carer, Vera. 'Then I'll write up the notes and check the medications out, if you'd like to come and check them with me?'

She got a nod from Vera. 'I'll just go and check on Mr. Smith, he gets restless this time of the morning. Won't be long.'

Left alone in the office, Alexis pulled the first file towards her. Not that there was much to write, 'Good night, pu'd x 3, settled well each time afterwards.' She muttered the words as she wrote them. The notes were all much the same, varying only in the number of times the patient got up for the loo, whether they had opened their bowels as well, and if they had asked for an extra sleeping tablet or pain relief.

She spent a little more time over Mrs. Jones' notes. 'I feel that this lady would benefit from some grief counselling. She is showing signs of depression in excess of that which might be expected from her recent bereavement.' She sucked the end of the pen for a moment. 'She also shows signs of confusion. Could the day staff send off the fresh urine sample I have obtained to eliminate a UTI rather than grief?' Alexis sighed, it must be horrible to lose someone you've lived with for forty or fifty years, but even more horrible not to have had that closeness.

She wrote up Jimmy Young's notes as well, straining her political correctness to the limit. 'Mr.

Young has a tendency to use his hands rather too freely. New nursing staff need to be aware of this in order to take avoiding action.' She grimaced over the file and flipped it shut, sitting back. Jimmy Young had had a hand on her breast before she could stop him, and claimed he was just grabbing her for support. But the hand had lingered a bit too long for comfort. The carer had said he made a habit of it, but at ninety they felt it was a bit too late to do anything but take avoiding action.

She pulled the final file towards her, recording the vital signs. She hadn't liked Mrs. Bartholomew's colour and had taken her blood pressure. It had been on the high side, but she was on BP medication, and everything else had appeared normal. The elderly had multiple medical problems; few of them in this home escaped something. Arthritis, heart congestion, COPD; but then they were all old, and the body could only take so much before it began to fail in one area or another.

Alexis patted the file shut and got up, going into the small drugs room and beginning on the morning meds, putting them into little plastic cups for each patient where they were regular.

She went to the locked cupboard and lifted down other pills which had been prescribed as extras; mostly Antibiotics, some steroid cream for a nasty leg ulcer, extra pain relief for a laceration on an arm. All very normal for this type of patient and the nursing home. Vera came in and they checked those off against the chart before putting them into the relevant cups as well. 'I don't usually do this job.' Vera spoke as Alexis signed her name for the final time that morning.

'How do you manage?'

'We usually have two staff nurses on, but one's off sick and the other needed a couple of days off. She's done ten shifts in a row. She'll be back on Friday.'

Alexis nodded her understanding. Ten nights would leave her in need of more than just a 'couple of days off' herself. 'Thank you, you've made my shift very easy.'

'That's alright, ducks, it's been a pleasure, will you be back again tonight?'

Alexis nodded. 'Probably.'

'Then I'll see you then.'

Alexis went into the office again and began the handover to the day shift, passing on verbally the things she had recorded, and adding a little which couldn't be written because it was either speculation, or possibly slander in the case of Mr. James Young.

Two days passed in this manner with Alexis, sleeping during the day as best she might. Traffic, barking dogs, washing machines that were apparently going for walks in the flat above and small children seemingly being murdered in the roadway by tired mothers, all contributed to the daytime noise and her lack of sleep.

The fourth shift, on the Friday, was slightly different. To start with she hadn't managed any sleep at all during the day. The council had decided that since it was summer and there was more traffic on the roads they would just dig said roads up, and use Alexis's road as a diversion route. 'Wonderful.' she muttered to herself as she buried her head under the pillow, again.

She hadn't slept as the clock ticked around to midday. She rolled over in the bed and gave a theatrical groan as she looked at the clock on the side table. 'Oh, bugger.' She dragged her reluctant body out of the bed and went to the loo, making a face at herself in the mirror in passing. She was just washing her hands when the doorbell rang. 'Oh God, preserve me!' She went blearily eyed to the door.

Josh stood there looking at her immaculate in his consultant's suit. His hair was neat and his face smoothly shaved. 'What the hell happened to you?'

Alexis shook her head. 'Pardon.' She looked past him and down the road at the large haulage truck thundering passed, then held the door open and walked away.

Josh walked in and closed the door behind him. The noise diminished but didn't fade away. He walked down the hall following her t-shirt clad body into the kitchen and admiring the long legs on display. Alexis went to put the kettle on. Swinging around afterwards to look at her visitor, she said, 'Good afternoon, Josh.' as politely as she could manage, but she really hadn't the energy to spar words with him today. And certainly not when he looked so spruce and she felt like a dog's dinner beside him.

Cardiac Arrest

Josh looked her over, she looked exhausted and untidy, and beautiful enough to get his libido sitting up and begging. He had been to the house several times over the last few evenings, only to have the doorbell ignored. He had become increasingly anxious; worried about the way he had dismissed her. Now here she was, looking eminently bed worthy and unconcerned. His temper spilled over.

'Where have you been? I've been around here knocking on this door, only to be ignored, and now I find you in bed at midday. Is he here too?'

Alexis looked at him in total bemusement. 'Who?'

'Bloody Peter. Remember he kept you awake rolling on you?'

'Eh, Peter's at home.' She shook her head, what was the man talking about. 'He came by last week, we went home for a few days but he doesn't live here.'

Josh, his worst fears confirmed, backed away and came up against her kitchen stool; he sat down abruptly and with a thump, just glaring at her from chilly blue eyes, his hands balled into fists.

Alexis looked at him. He looked, she licked her lips, good, desirable, angry, she sat herself down on the other stool. 'Josh, what do you want?' She put a hand on his fist.

The answer, 'You.' didn't seem like a good one to say at the moment. Josh looked down at the hand resting on his. He looked past the hands to her legs.

The white lines criss-crossing the tops of her thighs were numerous and clear against the slight honeyed tones she had acquired from her days in Whitehaven.

He frowned, following the lines as they disappeared under the hem of her nightie.

Alexis, wondering at the sudden silence and stillness, focused where Josh was looking. She stood up, stepping back from him. Josh held her eyes as he too stood.

'When?' He nodded at her legs.

'None of your business. What have you come here for, Josh, because if you haven't got an answer, I suggest you go.'

Josh held both hands up in the peace sign. 'Right, none of my business.' He kept his eyes on her face. 'I came around to apologize, I was worried and shouldn't have spoken to you the way I did.' He swallowed. 'My marital problems were colouring my attitude towards you.' He lowered his hands. 'I was worried when I got no reply. I went to the agency but they didn't seem to know where you were?'

'Well, they wouldn't. I didn't tell them.' Alexis felt her lips twitch. 'I've been working nights.'

'Ah. That explains the... ' He waved an expressive hand at her attire.

'Yeah, just wait a mo',' Alexis brushed past him and went towards the door, 'two shakes of a lamb's tail.' She disappeared.

Josh, left in the kitchen, sat down again, shaking his head. He shouldn't be here, jealous fool that he was. He didn't move though; he watched the door, waiting for her return.

Alexis came back in wearing jog bottoms and top in a nice shade of powder blue. 'How is Emma?' She spoke as she walked barefoot across the kitchen floor and went to make tea. She held a teabag over the pot and raised an eyebrow.

'Yeah. Please.' Josh watched her going about the humdrum task without speaking.

'Emma?'

He recalled his wandering thoughts. 'Emma is... ' he paused, 'Emma is alright, but her kidneys are failing.' He sighed. 'This last bout of pneumonia has knocked her for six. I wondered if I could persuade you to come and visit. She keeps asking where you are.' Alexis set a mug in front of him.

'I'm not sure that's such a good idea, Josh. She probably associates me with medicine and treatment and pain.'

Josh looked at her face, reading the indecision and fear there, but totally misinterpreting it. 'Are you sure those are your reasons? Em' misses you. I promise to keep my hands to myself, if that's any incentive.'

Alexis, reflecting that actually it was more of a disincentive feeling the way she did about him, firmed her lips. 'Yes, I'm sure about my reasons, Josh.'

Josh wasn't going to plead, she had 'Peter back home', he had no rights here. Whether he wanted them was another matter. He stood up, ignoring his untouched drink. 'I think I'd better go, I'm glad you're alright. Where are you working by the way?'

'A nursing home.'

He raised both eyebrows but said nothing for a minute. 'The job offers still open if you want it.'

'No, thanks.' Alexis looked up at him. 'I'm going home soon.'

He nodded. 'I'll see you around. Get some sleep.' He walked out, leaving Alexis confused.

'What a strange conversation. We never seemed to say what we meant.' She shook her head and went back to bed, sitting up to finish her tea and then sliding down and praying for sleep.

Chapter 9.

EXHAUSTION EVENTUALLY BLOTTED OUT the sound of the road, but the unremembered dreams made it a less than peaceful experience. She awoke heavy eyed, and vowed she would take another couple of days off after tonight's shift. Four nights was plenty, how that poor staff nurse had managed ten nights beat her.

The home was quiet and peaceful when she arrived. The familiar smells of talc, old people and dinners, wafted to her on the warm evening air. She was surprised to find another RN on duty as well; she'd forgotten that one of the regulars was due back.

'Hi, I'm Moira.'

'Ah, yes. Vera told me. I've got to admire your dedication.'

'Yeah, more like desperation!' Moira chuckled as she led the way into the office. The two women settled down to read the notes through after the drugs round, without any worries, exchanging comments and information.

Apparently she'd been right about the UTI. Alexis noted that Mrs. Jones had been started on Trimethoprin, for a 3 day course, that morning, she'd keep an eye out for symptoms of sensitivity; sometimes it made the patient's mouth sore. She gave a chuckle when she got to Jimmy Young's notes. One of the day staff had written, 'Beware octopus tentacles'. Not perhaps politically correct but everyone would know what it meant. She flipped through, making notes of any changes of medication or needs.

At four in the morning she set off to do a round of the sleeping residents while Moira made tea for them both. Mrs. Phoebe Bartholomew was sitting up in bed. She was a big woman, rather jowly, with protuberant eyes. At the moment they were filled with a species of panic.

'Oh, nurse, I do feel, ill.'

Alexis sat on the side of the bed, taking one of the chubby hands and setting her fingers over the pulse. 'Tell me what the problem is?'

'I should never have had the trifle, nurse, but I can never resist sweet stuff.' She tried to smile, but her face twisted in a grimace. 'I've got indigestion that bad.'

Alexis, busy monitoring a pulse which was bounding along like an antelope fleeing a lion, nodded. She didn't think it was indigestion, but it might be. 'When did it start? Had you been asleep?'

'No, I couldn't sleep a wink for the heartburn, and then the indigestion started. Oh, it does hurt.' Alexis nodded. 'I'll get you some tablets, but first I want to take your BP.'

'Oh alright, nurse. But I'm sure it's the trifle.'

Alexis walked quickly down to the treatment

room and brought back the sphygmomanometer. 'Right, I'll just wrap this around your arm and check it out.' She pressed buttons and waited for the machine to register. 210 over 137. That was not good. In fact she was sure that Phoebe Bartholomew was on the verge of, if not actually having, a heart attack.

Alexis rang the bell at the side of the bed and waited for one of the carers to appear. 'I would like you to phone for an ambulance for me, tell them we have a suspected ongoing MI here, and give them Mrs. Bartholomew's details. Then could you please ask Moira to bring some indigestion tablets.'

She turned to the frightened woman. 'I'm going to send you to hospital, just to be on the safe side.' She smiled. 'Let's be sure that your indigestion is only that. OK?'

'No, I don't want to go, not on my own.' She started to cry. 'Can't you come with me, nurse?'

Alexis frowned but before she could answer, Moira came into the room. She gave a wry smile. 'Welcome to my world. Here you are, Phoebe, some Gaviscon, that should settle the indigestion, and if the pain goes away we've lost nothing, and you get to see some handsome doctors. Ambulance is on the way.' She looked at Alexis. 'Could you act as escort? Would you mind? We can manage, and it would be better to send you and me stay here.'

Alexis nodded. 'If you're sure.'

Moira nodded. 'I'll get her notes for you.' She looked at the elderly woman. 'OK, Phoebe. Alexis will go with you and see that you're alright in the ambulance.' She disappeared through the door and Alexis patted the hand still gripping hers.

'There, all sorted.'

Alexis waited until the paramedics arrived, and then fetched her bag and jacket before climbing in the back with Phoebe Bartholomew. 'All comfy. How's your pain now?'

Phoebe shook her head laying back against the hard couch with an aertex blanket over her and straps to keep her stable for the journey. 'It still hurts something chronic, all down me arms. I'm never touching trifle again!'

Alexis laughed, but she was monitoring the ECG machine that had been applied after they had the elderly woman aboard the ambulance. 'We can give you something for that pain is that alright?'

'Oh, just make it go away, nurse.'

The paramedic nodded at Alexis; he already had a cannula ready to insert and got busy. They checked out an ampoule of Morphine and shot 5 ml into the chubby arm and then he gave a rap on the interconnecting door. Take it away, Sal.'

The short journey was uneventful. Phoebe Bartholomew slipped into a drug induced sleep within minutes. The Paramedic kept a careful eye on the BP and O_2 levels and Alexis sighed with relief when they arrived at the big double doors to A&E.

Six in the morning is not an ideal time to be arriving at A&E. Staff shift changes, handovers, people falling over as they get up, children with mysterious stomach aches that might prevent them from doing their homework or cleaning their rooms, asthma patients whose inhalers just aren't working after a night laying flat in bed. It's a busy place.

Saturdays are even worse; people who haven't made it to the doctor all week, but now decide they must have coughs, sniffles and rashes looked at and who can't get an appointment with their own GP, turn up at the A&E waiting room, and demand to see a doctor.

The situation this Saturday morning was made worse by a lorry and bus full of night shift works hitting head-on at a city junction, causing several other cars to hit them as they frantically tried to avoid the pile up and didn't succeed. The place was awash with trolleys and the walking wounded.

Alexis found she was being left in charge of her elderly patient with no chance to get back to the home. She settled down next to the hard couch and kept watch as the machines beeped their way through a regular check of pulse, BP and O_2 saturations.

Phoebe Bartholomew was a sick woman. She surfaced as the morphine wore off. 'Oh, where am I?'

'It OK, you're in hospital. How's the pain? Can you give me a score out of ten? That's the worst.'

Phoebe panted a bit. 'Bout a seven, maybe eight, nurse. Oh I do feel sick!'

'OK, we'll give you some more pain relief. Just hang on a minute.' Alexis found a vomit bowl on the shelf and then disappeared outside the curtain and went over to the desk. 'Can we check out some more morphine?' She gave a smile. 'And maybe some Maxalon, otherwise she's going to throw up on us.'

'Sure, just give me a minute.' The night duty nurse looked across the space and hailed a familiar figure. 'Hey, Josh, it's about time you turned up.' He grinned at Alexis. 'Josh will do a quick exam; we're rushed off our feet.'

Josh squashed the feeling of delight at seeing Alexis, albeit a very formal Alexis from the last time he'd seen her; this was neither the time nor place. He came over. 'I came as soon as I could, but for some reason the traffic is stalled in the city centre.' He offered a wry grin to Bill Sharpe. 'Hello, Alexis.'

He looked at Bill Sharpe. 'So, what you got for me that I had to be dragged out of my bed?'

Bill nodded at Alexis. 'Got a possible MI in cubicle four, and when you've done that, there's a lorry driver with chest pain in cubicle six. Not sure what the story is there; he's only just arrived, we haven't even triaged yet. I called you on the paramedics say so.'

'Alright, lead me to it.' He followed Alexis across the room and behind the curtains.

'I was going to get some more pain relief, but it's probably just as well you seeing her unsedated.' She smiled at Phoebe. 'This is Mrs. Phoebe Bartholomew, aged 87, known cardiac history. BP at six this morning 210 over 137, not noticeably reduced, chest pain radiating to the shoulder blades and left arm. ECG indicates ongoing MI. Pain at seven.

Josh gently shook a hand. 'Hello, I'm Josh, a cardiac consultant. Let's have a listen at that chest of yours and see if we can't make it easier for you.' With Alexis lifting nighties and shifting blankets, Josh listened to a chest that was wheezing at every intake. Alexis flipped the sheets about and he pressed lightly into each upper foot. 'Pitting oedema. Fluid overload?'

'That's what I thought, yes.'

'Right, let's get her started on some IV Lasix, see if we can't dry you out a bit.' He smiled at Phoebe. 'She'll need warding. Back in a minute.' He disappeared through the curtain and returned promptly with a plastic dish. 'Morph and max. Bill said you'd asked for it and the Lasix.' He looked at Alexis, got her nod and shot the dose home. 'You'll feel better in a minute.' He stood watching as the pain relief took effect. 'You can come and help me, Alexis. She'll sleep for a bit and they've enough to do here without dragging someone away from their work.'

Alexis opened her mouth then closed it again, what he said was correct; it was just the high-handed way he said it that got to her. She cast a look at Phoebe Bartholomew, who was snoring quietly, tucked the covers around her more securely and followed Josh out of the cubicle.

'Hello, *Cariad*.' Josh grinned down at her. 'I knew I'd get you working for my team if I waited long enough.'

'Josh.'

'I do like the way you say my name.' He walked through the chaos of patients and over to the sinks and washed his hands, then stood aside for Alexis to do the same. 'Now for cubicle six. Let's see what you make of that.'

'I'm not a doctor, or a consultant, for that matter.' Alexis spoke a tad peevishly. She was tired and hungry and she didn't understand why Josh was in such a good mood.

Josh didn't understand his mood either. He'd gone away the day before feeling more than a little depressed. It wasn't in his nature to poach on another man's preserves and he did know about Peter. But he had felt so happy when he saw her standing in A&E that he couldn't keep the bubble of joy down.

He led the way to the cubicle and the middle-aged man half sitting on the hard bed. He was bent over, clutching himself under his ribs. His right arm was swathed in a BP cuff and a pulse oximeter was attached to the left hand, Josh introduced himself while he observed the grey colour and the tension in the shoulders. 'What's your name?

'David Bowes.' It was huffed out between grunts of pain. 'Called me Dave.'

'Can you tell me what started this pain?'

'I dunno, Doc. I was feeling a bit sick like, and then I went all clammy and a bit fuzzy. I tried to get the rig to the side of the road, but I couldn't pull hard enough, and the next thing I know I'm coming around with a paramedic flashing a light in me eyes. He said I'd hit a bus, can you tell me if I killed anyone? Dear God, don't let me have killed anyone!' He let go of his chest to grab Josh's wrist and look up at him.

'Indeed you did hit a bus, but there were no serious casualties. Shock, bumps and bruises, you were obviously slowing down when you hit. Try to relax. I want you to slide down the bed a bit for me, so that I can listen to your chest and you can show me just where the pain is, OK?'

Josh watched Bowes ease himself down against the single pillow.

'Can you straighten your legs a bit?'

'It's better if I don't.'

'Have you been sick?'

'Nah, feel sick, can't seem to actually get it up.'

Josh nodded. 'Where else is the pain?'

'It's in me back and me arm. It's a heart attack init, Doc?'

'Let's find out shall we?' Josh glanced at Alexis. 'Can you just undo things?' He was all professional doctor now and Alexis responded to the tone. Undoing buttons and exposing a rather hairy chest to view, the chest had paper stickers in strategic areas. Josh noted them and looked at Alexis, 'What's the readout say?'

She looked at the paperwork on the side, 'Normal sinus rhythm, tachycardic, elevated BP'

'Let me just have a listen here, Dave.'

Josh placed the bell of the stethoscope over the chest and listened intently. 'Hmm. Can I just have a feel of your tummy?' Dave tried to straighten out a bit but presented a hard surface to Josh's enquiring hand. 'Have they given you any pain relief yet?'

'No, medics said it was better presentation, whatever that means.'

Josh nodded. 'Let me relieve your mind, I don't think you are having a heart attack.'

Dave shook his head. 'I heard about all them symptoms; chest pain, left arm pain, heart going like the clappers.'

'You have got pain, but I don't think it's your heart that's giving you it, and extreme pain causes your body to produce adrenaline and that causes your heart to 'go like the clappers'. Wouldn't you agree, nurse?'

Alexis nodded, giving Dave a smile.

'What would you say we've got here, nurse?' Josh kept his eyes on Dave as he spoke monitoring breathing and skin colour.

'I think it might be your liver, pancreas or stomach. Your vital signs don't indicate a heart attack.'

'I would agree, I'm going to get you booked for an ultra sound to see what's causing all the pain. But I'll also go and get something to get rid of it for now. OK?'

'If you say so, Doc.' Dave relaxed slightly and Josh smiled. Half the tension was apparently due to fear of a heart attack. 'If you could just check it out with me, nurse?'

Josh smiled at Dave and then they left the cubicle and walked across to the drugs room. 'So, my non-doctor or consultant, what did you make of that?'

He held a vial of pethadine up and Alexis checked it before he broke the ampoule and began drawing it up.

'I think he's either got a stomach ulcer with referred pain to the back, or pancreatitis, or a very nasty case of indigestion.'

'Yeah, that was my take. But if he passed out it's more likely to be the first two than the last. We shall see.' He gathered equipment to insert a cannula. 'I'll give this subcut and then get a cannula fitted. You'd better nip in and have a look at Mrs. Bartholomew while I do that. It might be an idea to get her catheterized as well.'

'It would certainly make her life easier, while we dry her out. And fluid balances?'

'Definitely.' Josh nodded, picking up his plastic dish. 'Meet you back here in twenty minutes.'

Alexis, gathering equipment to catheterize, from a place she didn't know her way around, muttered a few rude words about know-it-all consultants. She pushed a trolley across the room to be briefly stopped by Bill Sharpe. 'Everything OK?'

'Fine. Er, you do realize I'm not on your staff?'

'That's alright, Josh vouched for you, half the staff on duty aren't supposed to be here; they came in when they heard about the crash on the local news.' He glanced around. 'It's thinning off now. How's our lorry driver?'

'Josh is with him, he doesn't think its heart, and he wants an ultra sound doing ASAP.'

'I'll give them a ring, get things set up, the

quicker we can get them out of here and onto wards or sent home, the better.' Bill walked over to the main desk and Alexis carried on to cubicle four.

Phoebe Bartholomew was dozing nicely, but stirred as Alexis came through the curtains. 'How do you feel now?'

'Not as bad, nurse, but… ' She lowered her voice, 'I do want a pee something dreadful.'

Alexis nodded. 'That's the medication the doctor gave you, it shows its working. He's asked me to put in a catheter; will you be alright with that?'

'I had one of them with the last baby. That was many moons ago.'

Alexis smiled. 'We've come on a bit since then. They aren't as heavy, and you can carry the bag a bit more easily, but for now we just want to see how much is going in and how much is coming out.' Her lips turned up.

'Alright, dearie, if that's what you have to do. Doctor knows best?'

Alexis sniffed; she privately didn't think that was always true, but in this instance she thought Josh had called it right. 'OK, so if you'll lay back and let your legs flop, I'll get it organized for you.'

'Think of England eh?' Phoebe managed a chuckle as she arranged her legs to allow Alexis assess to her nether regions.

Ten minutes later Alexis was back in the dressing room, having tidied away her equipment, and was busy washing her hands.

'Ah, there you are.' Josh appeared at her side, making her jump. 'I've got a nice little head wound for you to stitch. You can stitch can't you?'

'Yes, Josh, I can stitch, providing it doesn't want numbing.'

Josh frowned. 'OK I'll shoot in a bit of Lignocaine and you can do the deed while I have another look at Mrs. Bartholomew. Got her catheterized have you?'

Alexis looked at him in exasperation. 'You asked me to do that, sir.' She sniffed.

'Ah, I wondered when you would slip up.'

'Eh.' It was all Alexis managed to say before a pair of arms circled her and Josh kissed her briefly but very thoroughly. 'You have been warned.' He grinned and walked out of the room.

Alexis stood glaring at the swinging door for all of thirty seconds. Bill, coming in, asked her if she was alright twice before she focused on him. 'Oh, oh yes, I wanted the Lignocaine.'

'That drawer there.' He nodded, took a stack of paper bowls from a cupboard and went out again.

Alexis muttered to herself as she set up another trolley with needles, gut and the lignocaine. What was the man playing at? One minute he was all professional doctor, the next he was kissing her socks off. She couldn't cope with the mood swings of the man, she thought, as she pushed the trolley and walked out of the room. Josh hadn't even told her which patient she was dealing with.

She looked around and spotted him emerging from cubicle four. 'Come on, Alexis, times a wasting.' Alexis sighed; what she would give for a cup of tea! She pushed the trolley over and then through another set of curtains. 'This is Miss. Elizabeth Graham, her head made contact with a shard of window pane. Nurse is just going to stitch it for you, and then you can go home.'

Miss Graham had an abundance of peroxide blonde hair and a very pretty face. The deep cut was half way along the side of her skull. Josh eased the hair away and shot numbing Lignocaine into the site and then, smiling, backed out. 'He's handsome isn't he, like on the telly, said it wouldn't leave a scar, clipped the hair so's it would fall over the spot and grow out.' Elizabeth Graham looked at Alexis. 'I bet you nurses chase him.'

'Not me, I've got more sense.' Alexis grinned. 'I'm fancy free and I intend to stay that way. Now let's have a look at this cut, it should be fairly numbed now.' She gently felt along the edges. 'Feel anything?'

'Nope.'

'Good, then 'let us begin' as my foster mother used to say.'

Josh, standing outside the curtain looking for the next patient, put his head on one side. He hadn't intended to listen, but it was very difficult not to hear what was going on behind that curtain. What did she mean she was 'fancy free'? Was she just putting a patient at ease, or did she really mean it? Foster mother, maybe she had a few hang-ups he needed to know about? He moved away, frowning to himself. He hadn't been able to resist that kiss either. She had looked so damn beautiful standing there.

Alexis came out of the cubicle, having finished her stitching, and talking about the latest fashion in boots as a distraction for her patient. She wheeled the trolley back, cleared away, and went to check on Phoebe Bartholomew. The porters were preparing to take her upstairs to the cardiac ward. 'I'll come up with you and see you settled in, shall I. Then I must let the home know what's happening to you, and they can get someone to bring you some clean clothes and things.'

Phoebe talked to her in a slow, dozy kind of way, as they got her into a bed and the day staff came to introduce themselves. Alexis said goodbye and made her way back down to A&E. She supposed she would have to get herself across the city and retrieve her car from the nursing home car park. But first she'd give them a ring and let them know what was happening.

She stood at the desk in the A&E, leaning against it as she waited for the phone to pick up at the other end.

Josh, observing her, saw the sheer weariness in every line. 'I'm a selfish bastard.'

He muttered the words and startled a young nurse passing him on her way to deal with a patient. 'Sir?'

'Nothing.' He offered a smile and then walked across the room, reflecting on the fact that he'd felt absolutely no desire to kiss that nurse for calling him 'sir'. His lips tipped up at the corners.

'I'll come back during today and get my car if that's alright with you? I'll let the staff know that you'll be in with her nighties and things. Thanks.' She put the receiver down and turned as Josh reached her.

He put an arm around her waist. 'The rush is over and you need to go home, Lexy. You look dead on your feet.'

'Thank you, kind s... ' Alexis stopped herself just in time, as she saw the gleam in his eye and felt his arm tighten slightly. 'That's not exactly a compliment, Josh.'

He shook his head. 'I forgot you'd been doing nights.' He shrugged. 'Come on, I'll give you a lift.'

Alexis frowned.'

'All I'm doing is offering a lift. I promise.'

'Alright, Josh. I was wondering if I had the energy to get home or if I should just crawl into a cubicle and pull the covers up.'

'Nah, the beds are much too hard.' He kept the arm in place as he guided her through the throng, allowing her to gather her jacket and bag from the rest-room before urging her into his Jeep Cherokee and watching as she buckled up.

She was asleep before he'd manoeuvred the vehicle out of the courtyard. He whistled tunelessly under his breath as he drove to his own home. She was going to be mad at him, if she could wake up enough. But he didn't care.

Chapter 10.

JOSH PULLED UP OUTSIDE his house with a thoughtful expression on his face. His passenger still rested in the arms of Morpheus. Her sleep had been undisturbed by traffic noises, and then the cessation of noise as he switched the engine off. He looked across the seat at her. What had he been thinking? He couldn't just kidnap a young woman and take her home like a stray pup.

He leant forward to turn the engine back on as Alexis stirred and open her eyes. She looked about at the faintly familiar street, then sat up and shook her head slightly. 'Josh?'

'Sorry. I'm sorry, Alexis, you looked so peaceful, I didn't want to disturb you.' He looked out of the windscreen and then back at her. 'I had this mad idea that if I could take you back to my house we might finally talk to each other. We seemed to be muddling along but never really understanding what we're both saying to each other.'

Alexis nodded sleepily. 'I know what you mean, but I'm too damn tired to talk.'

'Your room is still available. You could get a decent sleep here. You won't sleep with all the traffic going past your flat.' Josh half smiled. 'When you wake up we could talk.'

Alexis bit her lip. 'I am so tempted. Yesterday was horrendous!'

'You can go home anytime. I'm not holding you captive, but... ' Josh turned and took her hand. 'Give me a chance to talk, Alexis. I've made such a mess of things so far.'

Josh let go of her hand and climbed out of the car, coming around and opening the passenger door. 'Come on, Lexy; get some sleep in a quiet bedroom. Joan will call you in plenty of time to go to work, I promise.'

Alexis shook her head. She shouldn't, she really shouldn't, but she was so damn tired.

Josh hid his pleasure as she got out and went with him into his house. He pointed with his chin to the stairs. 'I'll send Joan up to see you've got everything. Tea and toast in bed?'

Alexis grinned. 'Now you've persuaded me.' She climbed the stairs and walked along the corridor, turning in at the familiar bedroom and looking around, the bed was freshly made, the windows open so that she could here the soft murmur of Maria speaking outside, and the sound of the birds; it was bliss. She sank down on the bedcover and removed her shoes and jacket.

Joan came through the door. 'Well, look at you, my lamb. Here.' She proffered a voluminous white nightdress in softest lawn. 'Put this on and climb into bed. I'll just be a moment and I'll fetch you a cup of tea.' She disappeared again and Alexis, smoothing down the pretty lace and beribboned material, sighed. Then picked it up and rapidly undressed before donning it. She was asleep by the time Joan returned with the promised tea. Her untidy head of hair released from its band and aswirl on the pillow.

Josh came up behind Joan, who stood in the doorway. 'I told you. She's exhausted, Joan.'

'That's as maybe, Josh, but you shouldn't be in here.' She turned, shooing him before her. 'Go on, get back to work. I'll look after her for you.' She shut the door quietly and followed him down the stairs.

Josh spent an energetic morning in his clinic. Every so often he would pause while he thought about Alexis asleep in the bed. He smiled secretly and softly to himself. They would talk, he would find out how committed she was to this Peter. He might even steal a kiss if she was willing; after all she hadn't exactly slapped his face when he'd kissed her earlier.

The object of his thoughts was still asleep at lunch time when he nipped home to check on her and his daughter. He did no more than grab a coffee with Joan and shot back to work. If he could have foreseen the afternoon events, nothing would have pulled him away from the house short of an atom bomb.

Alexis slept until nearly four in the afternoon; she woke to find her undies, and the scrubs she'd worn to work the day before, freshly laundered and lying on the end of the bed. There was also a cosy looking man's dressing gown. She pulled it on and went down the stairs in the quiet house.

She peeped into the deserted sitting room and then headed for the kitchen. Its pristine whiteness was only matched by its emptiness. Alexis eyed the kettle and decided that she must have a cup of tea or die in the attempt. She was just putting water into the teapot when the doorbell rang.

Still half asleep, she went into the hall and pulled the door open. The woman who had introduced herself as Josh's wife stood on the doorstep with a stranger next to her. He gave Alexis the kind of look which made her check that the dressing gown was fastened firmly.

Both of them exuded arrogance and heady scent in equal parts. Alexis looked from one to the other in confusion.

'See, he's got a woman living here. Now will you believe me, he won't let me have her.' Lesley turned on the tears, turning into his hand-made suit jacket and sobbing noisily.

Alexis looked astonished. 'I beg your pardon?'

Lesley turned back. 'Look at her, she's obviously sleeping here, and he says I'm not fit to have my child. Well, I will have her; you'll see to it wont you, Allan?'

'Of course, darling.' They pushed past Alexis standing with her mouth open, and went into the sitting room. She followed them, totally bewildered as to what was going on.

'Where's my daughter?'

'I don't know. I've only just woken up.'

'See she admits it. She's sleeping here.' Lesley looked at her, suddenly cautious. 'You're not married to him, are you?'

'What? Who?'

'Josh.'

'No. Of course not.'

'Disgusting, what kind of a man has his girlfriend sleeping in the house during the day, God knows what they get up to, my poor darling is probably grossly neglected.' Lesley gave a theatrical shudder. 'And he won't let me even take her to the park, just a little outing, that's all I wanted.' She began to cry again so that Alexis, trying to explain her presence, was drowned out by the near hysterical sobs.

'Well, I shall have her, I shall. You'll get her for me, Allan, she shall end her days with me. How can he be so cruel; keeping mother and baby apart like this?'

'Look, I'm sure there has been some misunderstanding here.' Alexis held the dressing gown with one hand on the collar, and looked at the pair facing her. 'I'm a nurse.'

'Well, isn't that typical, dating a nurse. I bet he was doing it the whole time he was married to me. It's unjust the courts giving him care of my baby; he won't let me see her even. I told you, Allan, I came the other day and he took her up to the nursery and threatened to throw me out. He even had a man here to help him, a security guard.'

'It's true he had a guard for her, but you

probably misunderstood him. I'm sure he wouldn't keep you and your child apart, he's a kind man.'

'I bet you know just how 'kind' he can be.' Lesley all but spat the words at her. 'Take me away, Allan. We'll take him to court if we have to.' She turned and stalked out of the room her tears miraculously drying up. Alexis followed, her protestations that they should stay and talk to Josh when he came in, fell on deaf ears. The door shut with a bang.

Alexis, tea forgotten, went back up to her room to dress. It seemed she didn't really know this consultant at all. If his wife was making such claims in front of a stranger about his behaviour, maybe it was true. Maybe he did run after the nurses as she'd first thought. Well she wasn't going to be a scalp on his belt.

Alexis pulled a comb through her hair. She didn't know what to believe, but she wasn't staying here, not until it was all sorted out anyway. She went down the stairs and quietly let herself out.

By the time she'd retrieved her car, cancelled her job at the agency, and driven to Whitehaven, she was a mess of nerves, and tears.

JOSH, RETURNING AT FIVE, having left the clinic early, entered his home to total silence. He went first to the kitchen and, finding that empty and Marie Celeste-like, was just walking back towards the sitting room when Maria, Joan and Emma came in through the front door.

Joan all but whispered. 'We took Em' to the swings; she was getting noisy. I didn't want her to wake Alexis up.'

'We'd better wake her now or she won't have time to eat before she goes on shift.' Josh smiled. 'I'll go and knock on the door.' He suited action to words, taking the stairs two at a time. 'Alexis? Wake wake.' He pushed the half open door wider and looked at the empty bed. He glanced towards the en-suite, but that door was open too. 'Alexis.' This time his voice was considerably louder.

He came downstairs as rapidly as he'd gone up. 'She's gone.'

'Maybe she was worried about getting home in time for her shift.' But Joan frowned down as she released Emma from her push chair. 'There you go, darling.' She looked up at Josh. 'Though I wouldn't have thought...'

'No, me neither.' Josh went into his study, glancing around in hopes of spotting a note on his desk. He headed for the sitting room; only to find that as deserted as everywhere else.

'Daddy, where's Lexy?'

'Twp! Penntwp!'

'Josh!'

'Sorry, Joan, but I knew I should have spoken to Alexis. I asked her to come, I was foolish enough to expect her to stay, and I told Emma she would be here and now... , I need to find her.'

Joan looked at him. 'You need to calm down a

bit.' She glance at Emma, her smile all but gone as she watched the adults.

'Daddy?'

Josh throttled back his anger and picked Emma up. 'It's alright, Em', Dad's not cross with you. Did you have a good time at the swings?'

Emma nodded. 'Dolly come too. Me show Lexy?' She held the rag doll by its neck and dropped kisses on his cheeks.

'Lexy had to go out, Emma. Shall you go with Maria and have a drink of squash then.'

'Want Lexy.' The little face began to crumple up and tears pooled in her eyes.

'I'll find her for you, Em.' Josh smiled, fretting, but taking Emma through to the kitchen he helped get her bathed, read her a story, and settled her in her bed.

He was nearly beside himself with worry and having to throttle back his feelings was making him feel almost ill. He wanted to go and find Alexis. By the time he'd managed to visit her flat Alexis was long gone, which, considering the towering temper he'd managed to build over the last few hours, was probably just as well for them both.

ALEXIS WAS ACTUALLY REGRETTING her precipitate exit from the house. She had had time to think about the conversation, and something wasn't quite right.

'I don't know what to make of things, Mother.'

Mary sat quietly for once, not occupied with a child. All the foster children were now in bed and asleep. Alexis sat across the kitchen table from her, nursing a cup of tea she didn't want. 'I think I've made a mess of things.'

'Hmm, that's a start, recognising that you could be wrong.' Mary offered a half smile at the young woman sitting frowning at the table-top. 'You say his wife came in and claimed he wouldn't allow her to see this child, Emma. But what had he said?'

'He wasn't there, but he had said she could see Emma but not take her out of the house.' Alexis spoke slowly. 'Given that she is seriously ill and only just recovering from pneumonia and that her mother hasn't had much to do with her, that's a sensible precaution.'

'Mm, mmn.'

'She seemed to be egging on this man she'd brought with her.' Alexis frowned. 'She's really pretty, Mother. She's got lovely clothes. I was jealous.'

'So she's pretty and dresses well, so what, Alexis? You know that looks and clothes aren't everything. What else is troubling you?'

Alexis sniffed somewhat inelegantly. 'Yeah, but... I think I'm in love with him...' she gulped admitting it out loud was a bit different to just thinking it she discovered. ' She looked across the table at the sympathetic eyes watching her, 'and he saw the scars, Mother.' It was said flatly.

'Did he run screaming from the room,

repulsed by a few white lines?' Mary raised an eyebrow.

'No, of course not.' Alexis shook her head. 'But he knew what they were.'

'And? I ask again, did he reject you?'

'No.' Alexis fell silent after the one syllable.

'Some time you shall explain to me, how a child I've brought up, came to show a man, not her husband, scars, at the tops of her legs.' Mary gave a faint chuckle as Alexis gave her a startled look. 'But for now I think you owe the man an apology, you left his house with out even a thank you note, you know better than that.' Mary held up a finger as Alexis would have spoken. 'What's more you owe him the chance to put his side of this situation. It seems to me that you have run away far too often just lately.'

'Yes, Mother Mary.' Alexis looked, and sounded, about seven.

'Tomorrow you will go back to your flat, Alexis, and you will then find this young man and apologise and listen to him. I don't mind supporting you; I'm not going to hide you. Is that clear?'

'Yes, Mother Mary.'

'Good. Come and give me a hug. I'll not go to bed in anger.'

Alexis came around the table and Mary stood up. 'I love you; you know that, Lexy. I just want what's best for you.' She held Alexis's face between her two hands and wiped away a tear with a thumb. 'This is your home; I'll always have a place for you here. Now go to bed, darling, and if you love him as you say, isn't it worth sorting things out?'

'Yes. But I'm scared.' Alexis looked anywhere but at her foster mother. Then mumbled 'I love you, Mother Mary.'

'Scared is allowed, even good, it means you recognise the seriousness of the emotion. But running and hiding is not allowed.' Mary shook her head and patted her on the back.

Alexis gave her a hug and went up to bed. She lay for a long time thinking about the various conversations she'd had that day. In a muddled way she knew Mary was right, she owed Josh the chance to explain himself, she'd finally admitted to herself the reason she was running. She loved the man, and his daughter, and she was terrified of the pain of more betrayal and rejection. She turned over and thumped the pillow. 'Coward.' She whispered the words as she resolutely closed her eyes and sought elusive sleep.

MARY DOWN HAD WAVED Alexis away the following morning and then laid her plans. Carl and Peter would go with her that afternoon to Carlisle Centre. They did need some small articles of clothing, but that was really an excuse. She was going to be on hand if she needed to pick up the pieces. Eva could be picked up by Susan's mother and stay there for tea.

ALEXIS, UNAWARE OF THE plans being laid to protect her if need be, drove back to Carlisle feeling half-resentful, and half-angry. It was all Josh's fault that she had been scolded by her mother, it was all his fault that she had acted in such a silly way in the first place.

In the deepest corner of her heart she knew it wasn't really his fault, but this way she could build up a wall of protection against the forthcoming rejection she was sure was coming her way.

She pulled up outside her house and noted the Jeep Cherokee parked two doors up. She swallowed and got out of the car slowly. She felt ill, going hot and cold at the thought of the coming confrontation. She'd thought she could choose her own time and ground for this fight, but apparently that wasn't to be.

Josh got out of his car as soon as he saw her alighting, so they met on the doorstep.

'Alexis.' The tone was neutral if somewhat chilly.

'Josh.' Alexis was fishing in her bag for her door key and kept her eyes down. She glanced up at his face, and then quickly away. 'You'd better come in.' She seemed to be having trouble opening the front door and Josh watched in slight surprise as she fumbled to get the key in the lock.

'Here.' He took it out of her suddenly nerveless hand and inserted it, turning and pushing open the door.

Muttering, 'Thanks.' Alexis led the way inside. She dropped her overnight bag and shoulder bag in a heap on the settee and turned to face him. 'I'm sorry.'

Cardiac Arrest

She spoke as Josh did; only he wasn't apologizing.

'I have been going half out of my mind. Where the hell have you been? You disappear like scotch mist, then reappear without a by-your-leave.'

She backed away slightly in the face of the fury she could read on his face. 'I said I'm sorry.'

'And that's supposed to fix it is it? 'My daughter is dying; I want whatever she wants and needs. Is that too much to ask? I want the best. You ... I thought you were the best.' He poked a finger at her even as his face sneered. 'God help us, even Lesley is prepared to spare some of her precious time for the child, and she knows Em's only got months left. But you, you can't even stay to see her overnight.'

'But ... '

'I told you how ill she was; I told you she wanted you. But no, you have to run off at the first sign of suffering. I know what those scars mean, don't think I don't.' He pointed a finger at her jean covered legs. 'I admired you for choosing nursing; it's full of suffering, trauma, pain. I thought you'd overcome your own. Learnt to deal. But no, you run away. Well Emma wants you. I'll put up with you, because of that. And you, Alexis, will just knuckle down and put up with me.' He drew a deep breath a looked at her.

Alexis had grown whiter and whiter as he spoke. Now she put a hand out and felt for the back of a chair, lowering herself into it with the care of an old woman.

'What are you sitting down for? I've told you,

Emma needs you.'

Alexis shook her head, not in denial but because she seemed to have a buzzing in her ears. Josh, watching her, was about to launch into another tirade when the doctor in him took over. He caught her neatly as she slipped sideways and would have landed on the carpet at his feet.

Alexis was out for the count and Josh, feeling a rapid pulse, and a fever hot brow, raised an eyebrow. 'Bugger.'

He picked her up and carried her through the flat, looking for the bedroom. The tidy and single bed brought an unexpected uplift to his heart, even as he set his burden down. He had reached the stage of taking off her shoes and unbuttoning her jacket before she swam to the surface again. He was sitting on the side of the bed feeling her pulse.

'Josh? I feel most peculiar.' Alexis frowned at him, looked about, and then tried to sit up. 'What are you doing in my bedroom?'

Josh shook his head and gently pushed her back down. 'You, Alexis, have one hell of a way of stopping an argument. You also appear to be running a temperature. Stay where you are while I get my bag.' He stood up and left the room.

Alexis frowned, then pushed herself upright, swinging her legs over the side. The action had the world dimming around the edges. She was shaking her head and trying to get herself onto her feet when Josh returned.

'Don't you ever listen to me?'

He gently eased her down again, opened his bag, and took out a thermometer. 'Open.'

Alexis, about to protest, found the instrument popped into her mouth and Josh gave a slight smile. 'Close. Now since there are two fairly infectious diseases you have been working with I need you to answer some questions. Answer with a nod, *Cariad*.'

He took her wrist again. 'Been going to the loo, bowels OK?

Alexis nodded her head.

'Been sick?'

A shake.

'Coughing?'

Another shake.

'Peeing OK?'

Alexis nodded her head, feeling her cheeks warming, even as she answered him.

'I want to listen to your chest, *Cariad*. Alright?'

Alexis scowled, muttering around the thermometer. 'There's nothing wrong with me and what's a Cariad?'

Josh shook his head and pulled out the thermometer, read the result, and then pursed his lips. 'Normally have a temp of 39 degrees do you?' His hand moved from her wrist to her hand. 'You really aren't well are you? Undo your buttons; let's have a listen to your lungs.'

Alexis, felt the heat rising from her midriff and

then shivered as Josh carefully hoisted her chemise and began to listen to her chest in a very professional manner, asking her to breathe deeply and cough.

'You would seem to have a chest infection.' He smiled at her. 'Hell of a way to take the wind out of my sails.' He gently tapped the bell of the stethoscope against his hand. 'What's to be done with you, you can't stay here on your own can you?'

Alexis opened her mouth to ask why not, but never got the words out. He was pulling his mobile out and pressing buttons even while she struggled for words. He spoke into the receiver and Alexis closed her eyes in frustration.

'You, *Cariad*, are coming back with me; Joan will look after you. I haven't forgotten I want a word with you, but you are in no condition to argue.'

She shook her head. 'Emma. You can't risk taking infection into the house.'

'I suspect Emma is the culprit that gave you this bug. But she won't be allowed near you until I think you aren't any danger to her.' He spoke with his usual high-handed consultant's voice, and Alexis just shook her head and closed her eyes, she was feeling light headed again.

Josh looked down at her and then repacked his bag; he went out, glanced around the sitting room, picked up overnight and handbag and went outside, slinging them in the back of his jeep before going back into the flat.

As he went in he met a middle aged woman

with two children. The elder child was being carried, and Josh raised an eyebrow at the obvious disability; the other child was on a rein but clutching her hand. He stood back to allow her to enter.

Mary Down gave him a nod of thanks and turned towards Alexis' flat. He followed now, both eyebrows were raised. 'Lexy, I just...' she tailed off as she realized that not only was she not being answered, but she was being followed.

She spun around. 'Who are you?'

'Josh Blevins.'

'Ah. And where's Alexis?'

'On the bed.'

Mary narrowed her eyes; she went through the door and set Carl down on the floor, then gave Peter a push. 'See if you can find Lexy for me, Peter?' She stood in the doorway, preventing him from coming in any further.

'What do you want here?'

Josh scratched his chin. 'Lexy is ill, I was taking her to my house for my housekeeper to look after. I'm a doctor.' He nodded at Peter toddling back towards Mary. 'Peter you said?'

Mary gave a curt nod. 'What of it? What's wrong with Alexis?'

'I suspect pneumonia.'

'Dear God, the girl will be the death of me. No wonder she wouldn't eat breakfast.' But Mary was talking to herself as she headed down the corridor towards the bedroom.

Alexis awoke from a slight doze to find her mother and Josh on either side of the bed, looking down at her.

'Mother Mary, what are you doing here?'

'I came to use your bathroom, Carl needs changing. What have you been up to now?'

Alexis swung her eyes towards Josh. 'He says I've got a chest infection.'

Josh nodded. 'Mother are you? Any history of heart problems in the family?'

Mary frowned at him. 'Adopted, I can give you some general information but...'

'Person alive here.' Alexis scowled at them both; 'I can answer my own health questions.' She frowned at Josh. 'Heart problems?'

'Bit of a murmur, nothing to write home about.' He shrugged. 'I just wondered if it was genetic. I was wondering if our children would inherit.' He divided a smile between the two women. 'Now we've got that sorted out, I'll take her off your hands and get her some antibiotics.'

Mary nodded at him. 'You'd be that consultant.'

'Well, I am a consultant.' Josh spoke cautiously.

Mary gave another nod. 'I'll just sort the bairns out and get out of your hair.' She smiled at a totally dumbfounded Alexis. 'Trust yourself, love.' She bent and dropped a kiss on the hot forehead and left the room.

Alexis tried to sit up without much success, as Josh just leaned over and held her with one hand on her arm. 'What are you talking about, Josh? Genetics and children, indeed.'

Josh smiled softly down. 'I think I've got it all worked out now, but we'll talk about it when you can argue back.' He then scooped her up and walked out of the flat, shouting a goodbye to Mary on the way.

The next three days were a bit of a blur to Alexis. Josh came into the bedroom in the mornings, did a chest exam while Joan stood at the end of the bed. Asked some very doctor-like questions and then disappeared. But by the Wednesday Alexis was feeling not only better but frustrated.

Josh, coming in that afternoon, gave her a piercing look and nodded to himself. 'Yes, you're ready for that postponed conversation now.' He pulled up a chair and sat next to the bed, possessing himself of a hand, and then waited.

Alexis lay back against the pillows and scanned the very handsome face and the blue eyes watching her so carefully. She opened her mouth, and then closed it again before saying. 'Josh, I don't understand. Why did you think I'd run away from Emma?' It wasn't the question she wanted to ask, but she didn't think she had the nerve to ask questions about children specifically his and hers.

Josh gave a gentle squeeze to the hand he was looking at. 'I should have told you about Emma's mother, but no-one likes to admit they've failed and ... ' He paused, 'I've become a bit protective of my daughter, it's a cruel world out there.' He raised his eyes and looked at her pale face. 'Emma is ... I got married when my wife, Lesley, told me she was pregnant. She was, but Emma wasn't my child. Lesley couldn't handle a disabled child. She wanted Emma put into care. But ... ' he gave a wry smile, 'I loved Em'. It wrecked our marriage.'

'But if she'd been unfaithful...'

Josh shook his head. 'Takes two to keep a marriage going, I wasn't prepared to try. I just didn't love her; I probably wouldn't have married her if she hadn't said she was pregnant. And she probably wouldn't have married me if she'd known how much my bank balance was worth.'

Alexis shook her head, hearing the bitterness underlying the words.

Josh squeezed again to gain her attention. 'I brought my baggage to our relationship, thinking you might reject Emma too.'

'But she's a love.'

Josh nodded. 'But, you see, you kept running away. I was looking for reasons, even while I was falling for you.' His lips twitched. 'I thought you'd got a boyfriend called Peter at one stage.'

'Peter? But Peter's a baby.' Alexis shook her head.

'Oh, I know that now!' Josh drawled the words. 'Jealousy's a funny thing, you seize on the most obscure statements as to why people might not like you.'

'I did like you, only ...' Alexis paused, 'I'm a nurse and you're a consultant and, anyway, I've got my own baggage. And your wife is very pretty and she doesn't look as though she has any baggage at all, though when I saw her I realized she was a bit emotional.'

'When did ... oh when she came to call that first time.'

'Well, first and second time. She has a lovely figure, Josh.'

'Tell me about the second time, *Cariad?*'

'Second time?' Alexis frowned. She still wasn't sure about that word Cariad and it was derailing her train of thought somewhat as was the hand holding hers.

'Second time.'

'She came while you were all out; I was feeling a bit groggy even then. She came and, and, well she more or less said I was your girlfriend and she was going to prove you were an unfit father, having your girlfriend living in. She said she would get control of Emma, I couldn't have her using me like that.' Alexis sniffed. 'I don't think I was thinking very clearly.

'She even said she would be able to have Emma with her and her new husband all the time. She was going to take her from you.' Alexis looked at their clasped hands. 'And I was jealous too, of all the other nurses she said you'd got running after you. I'm not pretty and ...' With a sweep of her hand she indicated her legs hidden under the duvet.

'Ah yes. Your mother said I should ask you about that sometime. I told her it didn't matter, but she said best to ask and clear the air. As to my ex, Lesley was trying a bit of emotional blackmail with her new boyfriend, it seems he wants a family and she was promising to deliver a ready made one. However, she won't deprive me of Emma, and it seems she slipped up with him too. He found out she was going for an amniocentesis test. He doesn't hold with that. Apparently if you're pregnant, you're pregnant, no abortions for him. So why have the test. She's dropped herself in it good and proper.' Josh shook his head.

'The boyfriend threatened to take her to court over her unborn child and she rather revealed her true colours. He didn't know Emma had CF and Down's either and while he would have supported Lesley if she'd been genuine, he wasn't going to disrupt a dying child. He and I have had a nice little heart to heart. I don't wish Lesley ill, but she isn't going to hurt those I love.'

He grinned. 'That includes you, *Cariad*.'

Alexis shook her head. 'What does that mean? You used it when you spoke to Emma too.'

He grinned. 'Darling, just darling. He watched the pink filling her cheeks as Alexis looked down in sudden shyness.

'And here's another word for you, *'cusan'*.' He watched the blush for a moment, 'Repeat after me, *'Rho cusan i mi'*.'

Alexis shook her head. 'I'm not saying

anything I don't understand.'

'OK, I'll demonstrate. Give me a ... ' he leaned over and began to kiss her, *'cusan.'* He said the word as he finally relinquished her lips. He sounded as out of breath as Alexis felt.

Alexis leaned back against the pillows and shut her eyes as the world did a slow dance. 'I thought that was a *'sws'.*'

'Oh no, a *sws* is this.' Josh moved and gave her a kiss on the cheek. 'That's for children and aunts and sisters and brothers, you can give our children a *sws*. This is for people you are in love with.' He demonstrated a *cusan* to the satisfaction of both before sitting back.

Alexis, now rosy, said, 'In love with?' not sure if she was dazed by the kiss, events moving too rapidly or the after effects of pneumonia...but she hoped it was the kiss and what that meant.

'Definitely.' He watched her face, and her closed eyes. 'It's usual to reciprocate, if you can?' He took both hands, holding them securely, but he looked and sounded a bit afraid as Alexis opened her eyes.

'My father died when I was seven, my mother died when I was ten. I found her. I hurt so much. I was so alone and I was in a foreign country and no one loved me for me. I started cutting. It eased the ache. But then it would rise up again. It's like a drug. You have to keep getting a fix and you need more and more, to cure the pain.' She looked at their clasped hands. 'I won't need that drug anymore, I've got someone who loves me, and whom I love more than words can tell. I love you.'

'Thank God for that.' Josh brought her hands to his lips and kissed the knuckles. 'Emma's still going to die, *Cariad,* you know that. It will hurt. I need you, she needs you, will you make her happy for her last few months? Will you be her mother and my wife?' Can you bear that?'

'Yes, Josh.'

'And maybe have another baby someday?'

Alexis nodded. 'Then we can tell him about his big sister and how wonderful she was.'

'God, I love you.'

'I love you too.'

About the author:

The author began writing after employment in numerous jobs. Among other occupations there has been teaching, interpreting, nursing, stoker on a steam engine and shop worker. This variety has coloured the writing and informed the writer, as all lives do.

Married with children, the temptation to commit murder has been firmly repressed, especially when family life has intruded into the time set aside for the enjoyment of writing both murder/mysteries and romance.

The author has lived in a number of countries including England, Scotland, Wales, and New Zealand and travel, as they say, 'broadens the mind and the vocabulary'. If the occasional expression is new, the motivation and emotions of people are the same the world over.

Also by the same author:

Relative Dating. (2008)   ISBN 978 1 9997425 2 2
                             EBook ISBN 978 1 9997425 1 5

Tree Dimensional. (2009)   ISBN 978 1 9997425 5 3
                              Ebook ISBN 978 1 9997425 3 9

Grave Doubts. (2009)   ISBN 978 1 9997425 7 7
                           Ebook ISBN 978 1 9997425 4 6

Diverse Distress. (2009)   ISBN 978 1 912462 03 2
                              Ebook ISBN 978 1 912462 02 5

Smokescreen. (2010)   ISBN 978-1-912462-05-6
                          Ebook ISBN 978-1-912462-04-9

Collide and Conquer. (2011) ISBN 978-1-912462-07-0
                                Ebook ISBN 978-1-912462-06-3

In The Loop. (2011)   ISBN 978 1 8438670 2 9
Timeline. (2011)   ISBN 978 1 9997425 9 1
                          Ebook ISBN 978 1 9997425 8 4
Enter Two Gravediggers. (2011) ISBN 978 1 9034906 6 2
Disreputable Truth. (2012)   ISBN 978 1 8438682 9 3
Discarded Images. (2014)   ISBN 978 1 910077 13 9
                              Ebook ISBN 978 1 912462 00 1
Entrapment. (2017)   ISBN 978 1 9997425 6 0
                         Ebook ISBN 978 1 9997425 0 8
Primary Care. (2017)   ISBN 978 1 912462 01 8
                          Ebook ISBN 978 1 912462 00 1

Printed in Great Britain
by Amazon